Get Blissed
Sever the Ties & Liberate Yourself

Natasha Aylott

© 2015 Natasha Aylott

Birmingham, England, United Kingdom
www.getblissed.co.uk

E:Natasha@getblissed.co.uk | M: +44 (0) 7825808994

All Rights Reserved

The author of this book does not offer any medical advice or prescribe the use of any drug or any technique as a form of treatment for physical or medical problems without the advice of a physician either directly or indirectly. Therefore the information given in this book should not be treated as a substitute for medical advice; always consult a medical doctor. Any use of information in this book is at the reader's discretion and risk. Neither author nor publisher can be held responsible for any loss, claim or damage arising out of the use or misuse, or the suggestion made or the failure to take medical advice. No part of this book may be reproduced in any form by any means without the written permission from both the copyright owner and the publisher of this book.

ISBN-13: 978-1511531948
ISBN-10: 1511531940

For information regarding special bulk discount purchases, please contact 10-10-10 Publishing at 1-888-504-6257

Printed in the United States of America

Contents

Purpose	i
Dedication	ii
Testimonials	iii
Acknowledgements	vii
Foreword	ix
Overview	xi
Chapter 1: Love Yourself	1
Chapter 2: Acceptance	19
Chapter 3: Forgiveness — The Ultimate Gift to Yourself	31
Chapter 4: Stop Worrying, Stop Criticizing, Excuses Be Gone	43
Chapter 5: Affirmations & Thoughts	57
Chapter 6: Wellness — Body, Mind & Soul	77
Chapter 7: Educate Yourself	105
Chapter 8: Stop Watching/Reading Negative Stuff	119
Chapter 9: Awareness	131
Chapter 10: Take Full Responsibility for Your Life	145
Conclusion	163
About the Author	165

Purpose

My desire is to be the expert in De-Stressing and Alignment for Busy People, and to continually enrich the lives of others by inspiring and motivating them to step into their own magnificence.

My dream is to help sow the seed in the minds of everyone I am privileged enough to meet in my lifetime, in order for them to realise their own worth, accept it and embrace it. For those wonderful people, whose lives I touch in some small way, to then go on to realise their own skills and gifts, discover their dreams and shine like the bright unique stars that they all are. This is the most incredible journey you will ever take, because it is your journey. It is the story of your journey back to you. The Ultimate Body, Mind & Soul Workout.

By recalibrating your life, by doing the work, you become the change you want to see in yourself. Set your intentions at your highest self, for each and every area of your life. Learn when to say no in a loving way. Live your dream.

Dedication

I dedicate this book to my amazing inspirational Russian immigrant grandfather Alvian, whom I adored, my clever mother Sue, who was wise enough to realise that, in order for me to grow, I needed to be pushed out of the nest to find my wings on the way down. To my husband William, who was brave enough to take me on. Also to my incredible, magnificent children Harry and Seren, who motivated me to become a better teacher and mother. My beautiful daughter, Seren, my depth of gratitude goes out to you for allowing me to use your beautiful picture for the cover of this book. To my precious son, Harry, who never ceases to surprise and amaze me with his inventions, gentle maturity and insight. You both have such gorgeous, big personalities. Thank you for affording me the time to write this book, and allowing me to follow my Bliss.

Testimonials

"Thought-provoking, inspirational, motivational"
Jane Francis

"I really enjoyed meeting with Natasha. I found it very interesting and fascinating and this has certainly re lit the flame again for me. I am looking forward to now reading and watching a lot more on this positive way of life. I love the way Natasha is so enthusiastic about the subject she is teaching."
"Very enthusiastic and lovely and think you could help us no end."
Michelle

"After a coaching session with Natasha, a friend texted to say her husband had had trouble collecting money from a customer and so the morning after our session together she tried to ask the universe about it and lo and behold the man was driving behind her husband, unexpectedly, and flashed him to stop and gave him the full payment then and there!! "
Helen

"It gave me a lot to think about and I think Natasha is lovely. ...her way of seeing and dealing with things is amazing. She is a very inspirational person and pulled emotions out of us so easily. For the first time, though, I feel nervous about this journey. It's like I've only been playing and sitting on the fence the last 8 months and now it's serious... I have to have faith now and that's scary!!"
Sam

"I really enjoyed the evening. A couple of things Natasha said really hit home with me - about taking responsibility for our life (and I haven't really been doing that with my health) and about

only seeking happiness within (and although I know this I have recognised areas where I don't do this - again with food, I think food will make me happy and have been making unhealthy sugary food remain a part of my life as a result of this). The timing was great, 2 days later I went off on holiday where I was able to do lots of thinking. I ate much more healthily on holiday and made much better choices. It is a way of living and it incorporates a really holistic approach - yoga, meditation, affirmations etc. as well as lots of info on food. So if I crack my eating I'll thank Natasha forever because it's always been an area where I am weak willed!
Anyway I think Natasha was brilliant and I really appreciate the time she gave up for us. We would love to do it again. "
Helen

"I tend to take things in and then process them. I want to thank Natasha, as I always feel so confused and she helps to clear my mind and seem to make it so simple. She helped me realise now that I'm trying to do too many changes at once.
I always feel like devil's advocate and I always seem to be challenging the things Natasha says. I take in everything she says and I do get so much from sessions with Natasha. As an excuse, it's kind of the way I was brought up, to question everything and trust nothing; I am working on it though!! Please take this as a positive critique; it is wonderful that Natasha has so much passion for what she believes in.
Natasha really does have a gift and really helped inspire me, I hope that she will be very successful in her career as there are so many people that she can help."
Sam

"I pride myself in being structured, and process driven, but that also gets me caught up in the whole thing. Speaking with Natasha, reading her book, doing the short exercises she recommended has changed that a lot for me. I no longer fixate

on the structure and process of doing things, but enjoy the journey a lot more, I am not exhausted anymore, and more so, I don't drive people around me crazy..."
Naval Kumar

"Natasha is a very inspiring lady. Particularly her constant positive attitude and commitment to helping others are exceptional. She has certainly helped me look at things differently. "
Tia

"I have known Natasha in a personal and professional capacity for a number of years. Her positive attitude and enthusiasm in all aspects of her life are infectious traits to say the least. Natasha is goal focussed and a thought leader in her own right."
Alok

"Natasha is a wonderful support and ray of sunshine in my life. She has shown me ways to overcome struggles and challenges that come from the most positive and loving place.
She is one of these people that you are unsure how you never met before.
Natasha shares superb techniques and ways in which to focus your mind into a place that works for you.
Her smile is infectious and she is an asset to any person or group looking for a way to change their life in the most amazing way. I couldn't recommend her highly enough."
Jo Edwards

"To be perfectly honest, I did not know what to expect from my session with Natasha, so was a little apprehensive. However, she put me at total ease. Commencing this session with a meditation was totally relaxing and made me open my mind. Her r voice was warm and reassuring. Throughout our session, I felt that Natasha took me on many journeys. It made me think about my actions and feelings. It also taught me to stop, take a step back, question and examine myself.

I realise that yes everybody has health problems, and Natasha knows about mine. I felt that she took me deeper than this and helped me question a lot about myself and how I manage certain things.

If I was totally honest with myself, she made me realise that I had become stagnant in my life, self-pitying, feeling unsupported without any true friends and in an unnecessary rut. I realise that I have allowed certain circumstances to stop me growing and my life had no direction, going nowhere.

Natasha touched on many different topics, such as nutrition to the excess baggage that I continually carry around due to my negative experiences and vibes in my life.

What has this taught me?

I have now taken a step back and am looking beyond. I have many questions for myself and realise I must start my own journey. I must overcome my obstacles, let go of the "excess baggage" and find the right path for me. I know there is one and realise that I need to kick start this for my own well-being. Hopefully with a more open mind, I can learn to like myself, feel my worth and begin a new chapter in my life. I need to learn to trust again, be less judgemental and build my confidence which as late has had a real battering."

Caroline

Acknowledgements

The LOVE that started it all, inspired by Louise L Hay, the space created by Eckhart Tolle by opening up my heart, mind and soul that elevated me to levels I never knew possible. My mentors, friends and inspirational colleagues who I listened to, engaged with and collaborated with. Thank you to those I put the intention out to, to connect with, my amazing editor, book architect, as well as the incredible team of people around me who have held me safe in that space to enable me to be free to grow and develop.

Thanks to Raymond Aaron, Jayne Williams, Derrick Mills, The late and incredible Susan Jeffers, Louise L Hay, Dr Wayne Dyer whom I have listened to for days, whilst cycling, resting and sleeping, Deepak Chopra whose calming voice educates me, Ryan Deiss whose get-up-and-go inspires me, Clate Mask for his honesty and openness, Jairek Robbins for being so generous with his time and having the rare gift to be truly humble, fulfilled and a beautiful example to us all, Karl Dawson for his wisdom, Loral Langemeier for being a fierce female go-getter, Sir Richard Branson for showing me what a human being is capable of, Lord Sugar for his determination to make it happen, Desmond Stockdale for the smiles, Louise K Shaw, my longest standing, bravest, wonderful and wise friend, Naval Kumar for teaching me to be a better sage ... and many others.

Foreword

The author, Natasha Aylott, has beautifully and effortlessly broken down the complex barriers we all create in the world, and found a straightforward, practical and useable way to look at ourselves and the world we live in, in a way that's easy to understand.

She has overcome her own hurdles, struggled through her own difficult life lessons and developed straightforward steps that can be adopted by children and adults alike. When we commit to totally transforming the way we view the world, ultimately that's what we see. I was astounded at the level of intimate detail and knowledge shared in this book on the subject of Wellbeing. Natasha has a remarkable capacity for love, which draws the reader in to share the secrets of the universe. Imagine a world where every encounter is filled with delight, even if it is meeting someone for the very first time. Consider a world where we connect on such a deep level that our understanding of each other, nature and mother earth all conspire to help us. Visualise a world where no one is left out, a utopia where everyone is included. This is a world that is possible now. With the power of intention, if the whole of England decided at the same time to see the world as a peaceful, loving place, the whole world would have no choice but to respond. Love is gentle, unconditional, and yet the most powerful of forces in the universe.

This book opens the doors for every man, woman and child to learn and follow these easy steps to achieve great health in their lives; to be happy in the workplace and exist joyfully and harmoniously in the world. Trust this wise guidance, open your hearts and minds, let go and trust, and discover just who you really are and how very powerful you are.

Raymond Aaron
NY Times Best-Selling Author
www.aaron.com

Overview

This book was written for you, my lovely reader, to show you that each life is unique. To help you recognise that every one of us is a limited edition. Every person is important, and every one of us counts. Once you realise this, your world begins to expand. And my wish for you, in fact my deep desire, is that by sharing this journey with me, your world will become a little lighter, happier and more exciting. The possibilities for you will become endless, and hope will appear in your life.

When you operate from a place that is "heart centred" you can create an exceptional life for yourself. A life that is healed from the inside out. Learn to live at your highest self. Get Blissed is the most incredible journey you will ever take. The reason this is the most incredible journey is because it is YOUR journey. The magnificent and wondrous journey of YOUR life. Life is an adventure, a gift for you to enjoy, savour and have fun with. Life is like a great big playground, so try the swings. If you don't like the swings, then try the slide. Your life is especially amazing when you set the intention, place your order, don't take it all so seriously and enjoy the ride.

This book presents easy steps that you can adopt to change your life around. The tragedy is that no one taught you how, until NOW! Here are the steps, which I will walk you through later. They will empower you and enrich your life, giving you back a feeling of control, Bliss and freedom.

Here's a poem by a lovely singer/songwriter, Audrey Young:

That's me, Audrey chilling out with my best friend Cindy
What a ball we had, it was so bad
Went to see The Wedding Singer

OMG what a movie
One you all must see
Belly laughs you will get
I will put money on a bet
Book and go to see it
With friends
You will have a ball
So give your friends a call
One last thing to say
Have a wonderful blessed day

Written Monday 23rd February 2015

Step 1 Take Responsibility

Take responsibility for yourself. I mean total responsibility for everything in your life, 100%. That makes you accountable and in control of everything that happens to you, including what is going on in your body and mind. Don't play the blame game; you're in charge, you are the one in the driver's seat. By assuming full responsibility for your life and everything in it, you take back your magnificent power. You are awesome, amazing and unique. There is no one in the whole world quite like you. There will be no one in the future millennia who will be quite like you. You are a wondrous, spiritual being who has come to this place called earth to experience, learn your lessons and grow. To love, to laugh, to live, to connect and to share.

Step 2 Learn to Love Yourself

Warts and all. This has to be the main focus and the foundation from which everything else can be built on, and built to last. If loving yourself seems a step too far, then learn to like yourself first. You really are your own best friend; it makes perfect sense. You have been with yourself your whole life, you have come this far, you are amazing, unique and incredible; very well done. Trust in your inner strength. Be there for yourself when times are hard. When you truly learn to love yourself unconditionally, anything your heart desires, that is aligned with your soul, will follow.

Step 3 Fear

Most people are ruled by fear. Fear of failure, fear of succeeding, fear of loss, fear of being hurt or deserted, fear of being unloved, fear of loving, and so on. From an early age, fear is instilled in our very being, and keeps us trapped. Fear prevents us from getting hurt at times, but mostly stops us from living a full life. Fear also inhibits us from fulfilling our dreams, and fear represses our desires.

Step 4 Stop Worrying, Judging and Criticising Yourself and Others

Worrying makes no sense at all. It is such a waste of precious energy, and takes up head space. We are all different. What annoys you probably doesn't annoy the next person. You are not the authority on how a person must be, as none of us are the same. Don't waste your time being preoccupied and worrying about yesterday. That's gone, let it be. Leave it behind. There's no point in worrying about tomorrow, as tomorrow can take care of itself. Tomorrow hasn't happened yet, so leave your tomorrows to unfold.

Step 5 Get Connected

We are all part of the same collective energy, the universal source. We are all slices of the same pie, and we are all part of the same magnificent and amazing power. When you harm someone else, you harm yourself, because we are connected. Ask yourself this, why would you choose to harm yourself? Well, you probably wouldn't and therefore you can sensibly say that you could go through life without hurting another person. Now, this is the road to finding your bliss, to having joy and deep fulfillment in your life.

Step 6 Acceptance

In each and every situation you have a choice. Accept it or take action to change it. If you are ever in a situation where it seems you cannot do either, then surrender for the time being until you can. That time will come because nothing, even the bad stuff, lasts forever. When you look in the mirror, chances are even for the beautiful people who walk amongst us, there is probably something you want to change about yourself. Accepting yourself just the way you are is very powerful. Our bodies are just the vehicles we have been given for this journey through life. None of us remains young and gorgeous forever. Age and life affect the way we look and perform on a physical level. Learning to love and accept yourself is a crucial part of finding your bliss. You can eat and drink great food, and look after your body to give you the healthiest life. When you become comfortable in your own skin and can shout out "I am what I am" then joy will flow into your life.

Step 7 Forgiveness

I don't know about you, but when I first came across this particular word, it may as well have been an enormous scary monster. You may feel the same as I did; that there was no way you could bring yourself to forgive this person or that person. But the truth is, if you really want to set yourself free and live an authentic life, forgiveness is the only road to lead you there. It is an enriching and releasing experience too. Now, I'm not suggesting that you go down that dark and terrifying forgiveness road all by yourself; you will need two friends to tag along. Love and acceptance are always happy to help, and they will give you the strength to face the things you need to forgive.

Step 8 Affirmations, Thoughts & Feelings

Affirmations are simply positive phrases to say to yourself in your head that help you. They are useful because they help to calm the chatter, the monkey mind, the constant conversation that you have with yourself. Your thoughts become reality and most of your thoughts are the same as yesterday. Once you recognise this and accept it, you can go about making changes to the things you think about, for the better. When you add the secret ingredient of feelings and put an emotion to your thoughts, those thoughts grow powerful and manifest in your life.

Step 9 Love your body

Everything is either fear or love. Fear leads to Dis-Ease, whilst Love sets you free. When we learn to fully love ourselves and our body, what we put into it really matters. What we eat, the types of drinks we choose, how much sleep we allow ourselves to have. How much exercise we take and what type. Most of us lead busy lives, with no time to think about what is in our food, and sometimes no time for food at all. This is because there are many pressures and everyone else is doing the same.

So we don't question whether we are making the right choices for our bodies; we simply do what others do, I get it. Most people follow the crowd, pretty much like sheep. We stop questioning whether that's good for us because we assume that if our friends, family and work colleagues are working late, skipping meals and getting by on a shake and a snack, then it must be okay. What is required here is some sensibility. Rather than accepting what we are told, what others believe, each of us needs to make some decisions about what it is we want for us, our families, our community, and our world.

Step 10 Exercise

Do what you love. This doesn't need to be the Olympics, or even a gym membership. Just do what makes your heart sing. It could be walking in the beautiful countryside, taking in the smells of the farms, nature, wildlife, the freshness of the air. You might prefer to ski like lightning down the crisp sparkling white slopes, with your heart pounding in your mouth and adrenaline pumping through your veins. For you, it may be a gentle row in a wooden boat meandering down the river, listening to the trickle of the water shining in the afternoon sun, or zooming round the formula one track at a race course. Do you like bouncing up and down on a trampoline, without a care in the world? Whatever it is for you, that gives you that pang of excitement, like a hundred butterflies in your stomach, that enormous satisfaction, that's what you need to be doing on a regular basis. These are the things that take you to your Bliss.

Do you see where I am going with this? Life, you see, is an awesome gift, a journey of great adventures, as well as that of lessons to be learned. The lessons you learn add to the wisdom you can then teach to your children and share with others. But beware, there aren't any short cuts. This way of life must be a commitment to yourself and I promise it will result in a life of joy, resilience and happiness.

Step 11 Meditate, Mindfulness, Being Present, Follow Your Intuition

The whole point of meditation and mindfulness, although they are different, is they allow for you to stop doing and just be. You can learn quickly that just by altering how you breathe, you can calm down a racing heart, feel anxiety reduce and watch as feelings of anger dissipate. If you haven't tried these techniques before, I invite you to give them a go. . Mindfulness is incredibly powerful and in less than an hour, with simple guidance, you will find that even after the most stressful of days, you can feel completely relaxed.

Learn to be present and focus on the present moment. Our wonderful men actually find this much easier than women, who insist on multitasking as if their passport to approval in life is being superwoman. Being superwoman is not cool, so chill and take care of yourselves. Stop to smell the coffee, notice the beauty of nature, the patterns in the clouds. Learn to listen to your intuition. We all have that quiet inner guidance system, but for the most part, we're too busy to pay attention to it.

Step 12 What You Think, Read, Listen To and Say Makes You Who You Are Today

The thoughts you think are powerful. If you realised just how powerful your thoughts were, I bet you would be more careful of what you thought about. You are in the driver's seat, which gives you all the power. Now what are you going to think about?

What you read influences you. Scholars and academics study books that serve them. Books that give them more knowledge in the subjects of their choice. By the same token, the books you read define you. What do you read? The tabloids, fiction, romances, non-fiction, financial papers, medical journals?

What do you listen to? What does it say about you?

What words do you use? Are they self-defeating? Are they encouraging? Do they sound very much like the words your father or mother used to use?

Who are you?

I will hold your hand and take you through, in more detail, all the ways in which you can change your life to reach your BLISS!

Chapter 1
Love Yourself

Learn to Love Yourself

Love lights up the world. You are a spiritual being living in a human body. The road that leads to living a fulfilled and magnificent life is being in tune with both facets of you. Embracing the body, mind, soul concept is the only true path to balance, joy and harmony in your life. The whole world concept is one where everyone is included and no one is left out.

Love is powerful, it can conquer all. When you learn to love yourself, you cease the search for someone else to validate you. When you are loveable, you are loved. When you truly learn to love yourself, you are set free, your heart opens up and the most wonderful things start to occur in your life. You begin to uncover the real secrets of the world, and the universe is waiting to catch you, support you and carry you along, like a beautifully soft, warm feather down duvet, protecting you and allowing you to shine in all your glory. You learn to trust and rely on yourself more, and become stronger as a result. You learn to be heart centred. To live from that place of love. To radiate love in all areas of your life. To treat others with kindness, respect and honour. Every word that is uttered from your mouth becomes a powerful yet gentle manifestation of your very being.

Before you become tempted to stop reading here, filled with disbelief at the words you are reading, remember there's nothing new to what I am telling you. You have forgotten, that's all. You have never learned these secrets of the universe, because those who taught you have forgotten too. Did you learn at school how to love yourself? Doubtful. Were you shown the framework of what a deep meaningful relationship looked like? Neither was I. It is for us to share this knowledge with one another, to teach these amazing and wise ways to our children and to live by them each day of our lives. Everything I am teaching you is to encourage you to see that you already have this knowledge inside of you, and it is for everyone. There is absolutely no one in this entire crazy world of ours that is excluded from these ways of life. That's what is so powerful and that's what offers hope, joy, peace and total inclusion. This is where our greatest power arises from. The power to put the intention out there that we are all from the same source. We are all equal and we can all learn much from one another.

Love is everywhere you look. The beautiful, glowing, velvet pink and red sunset, the warmth of the sun cascading across the land, caressing the earth and lighting up the day. The sunset that shimmers, the deep, rich, fiery orange of the glorious sun that sinks down into the sea before lighting up another part of our world. The sun in all this time has never said to the earth "you owe me"; just imagine how powerful a love like that could be for you and me? To work in perfect harmony, to ebb and flow as nature does so perfectly.

The moon creates the pull of gravity that gives us enormous waves to surf on and play in. Was that an accident? No, these characteristics of mother earth, the elements, are all completely intentional. Sure, they have a purpose to fulfil that satisfies the scientist and astronomer. But they are there to enhance your experience, which is equally important.

The sun's job is to light up the whole world and heat the very earth you live on. The sun keeps the bodies of the reptiles warm, for just enough time to keep them basking and going about their business throughout the day. The sun and bees and rain help the incredible plants, gorgeous flowers and delicious fruit and nutritious crops to grow for us to enjoy. Does that happen by coincidence? The trees absorb carbon dioxide and emit oxygen for us to breathe; we breathe in that oxygen and give back to the trees the carbon dioxide. Is that a fluke? No, I don't believe so. It's a perfect collaboration between mother earth, nature and mankind. Did mother earth not give us pure water in the underground lakes and mountain streams to drink, bathe in and enjoy? Has Mother Nature not been relinquishing her abundance of treasures, from oil to diamonds, since time began? There is love everywhere that you look, and if you are feeling uncomfortable with this it's just because you have never stopped to look at the beauty and love all around you, in every direction you turn. When you look for love, you find love. Feast your eyes on the majesty of this wondrous, most majestic and spectacular planet with its blue and green swathes, visible from outer space. Love can conquer all. Love does break down the barriers and love is the most powerful emotion one can feel. A mother would walk over hot coals for her child; that's love. A man would walk into a burning building in search of a child that's not his own; that's love. A grandmother would literally lift the weight of a car to rescue a crushed individual; that's love. When you love unconditionally, great strength appears as if from nowhere. The universe supports us, life supports us and life loves us. When we are truly ready to see, our eyes open.

The 5 Cs Crucial to survival

The 5 Cs are a really easy way to remember why we are here. So here goes:
You are here to CONNECT with others, to
COMMUNICATE and
COLLABORATE, to
CO-OPERATE and to have
CONTACT with one another.

We were created and put on this earth to connect. When we connect, we open up. Fear keeps us hidden from the world. Fear prevents us from being honest with yourself and others. When we keep our feelings locked away from the world, it's like trying to keep a beach ball under the water in a swimming pool. Over time, the effort required to keep our feelings hidden puts pressure on our body. Eventually, all those feelings either erupt or we keep them buried so far down that they make us ill. What feelings are you keeping hidden?

We are designed to not just connect, but to share the skills we were blessed with through collaboration and co-operation. We are designed to communicate with each other. To recognise the talents that have been bestowed on us , to enjoy the experience here on earth and to learn our lessons. We learn our lessons or they keep presenting themselves to us . You may have noticed over the last few years that patterns keep presenting themselves in your life. The same results show up, even though the people around you at that time are different. You keep on doing what you have always done, and expect the results to be different. If you want the results to be different, change what you do, and the results will change too. That is what your lessons look like. When these situations no longer appear on your horizon, you have learned your lesson. And then a different lesson will come into view. This is how you develop and grow as a human being. When you feel off balance, alone or confused, it is often because you have become disconnected with yourself or each other. This connection is essential for your well-being and your very survival. When a tiny newborn baby enters the world, connection to their mother is their life line. However, without this most necessary human touch, without being held and cuddled, the baby withdraws and in some cases, life can literally disappear. Without human contact a baby is at risk of dying due to lack of human touch, in essence neglect. The absence of love, which is so crucial to survive, has profound and devastating effects.

The outcome and fallout on your body without love in your life manifests by making you ill. You need to connect with yourself, with each other, with nature and with the universe. It is when this connection is broken that you lose your sense of self and togetherness. You forget that life supports you and loves you. You start to feel alone and isolated. In time, you may begin to withdraw from other people, until in extreme situations you totally avoid others. Contact with another human being, sharing that energy that we are made up of, can improve your health as well as your happiness.

Have you ever noticed when you are in a group, it feels like there's more energy present? It may be the energy you notice is positive or the energy might be negative. Well, that's because what you can feel is the highly charged energy you and everyone else is made of. You feel this connection. As a writer and having run my own business for 15 years, there are many times when I have felt isolated and desired the connection and energy of others. Connecting with others energises you and opens up your heart. When you allow this to occur, the channel for love can start to flow. When you are open, you can reach out for this connection. It is why we are here, to connect with others.

For some of you, the thought of connecting with other people may make you feel uncomfortable. It feels difficult because of your conditioning, perhaps the way you were brought up. The environment around you also has a dramatic effect on your behaviour. The peer pressure to fit in, toe the line, be normal, and do what everyone else does. You try to do what your friends do, what your boss tells you, what society expects of you. It seems unnatural for you to reach out. And yet, you were created to connect.

Eyes are the windows to the soul. For this reason, some of you may feel threatened, not wishing to make eye contact with those around you. You might feel embarrassed to allow others in, to see your true magnificence. You may feel that you have nothing to offer. The truth is you all have much to offer. Over time it seems as though society has lost the skill of connecting on a higher level with other men and women. To be able to look into another person's eyes and on a deep level connect with them.

Have you ever been at a party or perhaps a conference, where you have gone up to someone standing close to you and shaken their hand? Well yes, I am sure you have. Did you really connect with that person? Did you truly engage with them? Or did it feel more appropriate to pull your hand away out of politeness? Did you not listen quite as intensely as you could have; did you slightly avoid eye contact for fear of feeling uncomfortable? Were you trying to think up a witty one-liner to throw back at them, instead of really listening to what they had to say? Next time you are in this situation, consciously engage completely with the other person; look into their eyes when you are speaking with them. You will be connecting with them on a spiritual, intellectual and physical level. Once you are willing to open your eyes and your heart, the energy between you is set alight and on a profound, unconscious level, you delight in that contact with each other. I dare you to try it next time and see how it feels.

Recently I met a man who reminded me of this deep connection, this gift we have to reach out on a higher level and connect. He was my teacher and I was reminded of the importance of this connection. Who will be your teachers, mentors and coaches? This is an important lesson to us all not to be too guarded, but instead let the light and energy flood in. Be sure you don't miss out on this amazing ancient gift your ancestors discovered and used. Unless you can get past your reluctance to connect, and accept this is why you are here, your life will feel empty. Embrace the connection.

Some time ago, I discovered that one of my gifts was to teach how others how to connect with themselves and each other. To start by opening up your heart and soul, to feel the amazing energy and love we all have. The sad reality is that, for most of us, the thought of sharing with others and baring our feelings fills us with dread. I am grateful to my own teachers for showing me the importance of having an open heart and soul. The reason we close our hearts is the fear of rejection, hurt or ridicule. When you learn to break away from the opinions of others, your heart will open all by itself. Remember that what others think of you is actually nothing to do with you, but more about what's going on with them, so make it none of your concern either.

You also have a choice. How will you see the world? As a hostile place or as a friendly place? Whichever you decide, that's what you will find. Because what you focus on comes into view. Most people don't realise this, until it's broken down into bite-size pieces and explained to them. For those who choose to see the world as a hostile place, you will find dangers and scarcity everywhere. You will feel unsafe, and ultimately that's what becomes your experience of life, only changing when challenged by you. You may have noticed that, even though a hundred people show up at the same concert, each of them has a different perspective. They are bringing with them all of the prejudices and beliefs they have collected over the years. One may report that the experience was fabulous, whilst another may complain it was dull. This experience of the same event is felt so differently by each of you because of your inbuilt filters. Each of you has different coloured filters, and this affects how you see the world; what it feels like to you.

When you choose to see the world as a friendly place, everywhere you turn, you find proof of this. Your experience will be positive and fulfilling. You will notice beauty and abundance all over the place, and you will find safety and kindness everywhere you look. For the people in this camp, the world looks like a happy, joyful, adventurous and beautiful place. Okay, I am simplifying it for greater impact here, but essentially, this is exactly how it works. In essence, the universe is here to serve and support us, so what are you scared of? Jump right in.

When you collaborate, you share the wisdom as well as the work. It makes perfect sense to work together. The word collaborate actually comes from the old Latin word "competere" which means come together. This translates to "compete", the meaning of which has become distorted over the years. Compete nowadays is used as a way to identify a winner, so far from its original meaning. By recognising a "winner" there also has to be a loser. This philosophy that we seem to live by actually divides us . It causes us to feel separated from one another. Separation and competition, as it's known today, leads to you not embracing togetherness, but rewarding individuality and independence. From this, disagreements occur, then fall-outs, then eventually wars. "No tree has branches so foolish as to fight amongst themselves", an ancient Native American quote.

Collaboration means to give the best of you and in return accept the best of others. It is perfect. In any group of people, there are so many incredible skills. Together, a collective can design, draw, plan and create a most wonderful building. Look at the Eiffel Tower. Just think for a moment of the hundreds of different skills involved. And yet if those skilled people didn't want to work together, if they were unable to see the end result and focus on the bigger picture in their mind's eye, that wonderful piece of architecture would never have come to pass. When you connect, collaborate and co-operate you become the very best of yourselves, and operate at such a high level that it flows. Let's learn from nature , the bees work in perfect harmony together. They all have their own roles to play and yet are consciously part of the greater wisdom, the collective wisdom to support and sustain their queen. By doing so they know their future is secure. Incidentally, the next time you see a honey bee, bless it, send it your love, because without these unbelievable insects we would have no fruit, flowers and vegetables. They are majestic, they are your allies. The ants are another species who work together in total harmony. They flow along as part of the whole. Much can be learnt from nature.

You were given hands and arms to wave and gesture, to write and hug. You were given a mouth and vocal cords to sing, speak, kiss with and yell . You were gifted two feet to dance upon. You were endowed with not just one, but two ears to listen with. You were given a brain to tie it all together; essentially you have so many tools through which to communicate with others. And yet, when was the last time you properly engaged your brain before you spoke? When you communicate, do you use your ears? Do you truly listen to what the other person is saying, or is it just noise? Are you too busy thinking about what to say in response to your colleague's sentence? You have been given so many incredible ways in which to communicate with others., it would be a travesty to waste them. You know how wonderful it feels when someone is actually interested in what you have to say. When they listen to you intently, when they give you their full undivided attention, it makes you feel valued, important, cherished. Once you become aware of this you can begin to make this a practice in your life.

Some of you may even be afraid of connecting in your own marriage. Contemplate why you may want to shy away from the person you love. This does beg the question why? Because of fear. Fear of getting hurt or feeling rejected. There are ways you can heal this part of your life at a time when you are both willing. When you purposefully send love to another human being, when you make that your intention, love will be there. Where there is no love, bring love, then there will be love. Love is an energy more powerful than any other. You can bless the rooms in your house; bless your car, your drive, your garage, your garden. You can send love to every area of your house. You can offer a smile that you hold a little longer than usual. You can put aside the ego of competition, or one-upmanship and allow yourself to feel peace and love. Try to recall the best time you had together and start the conversation with this feeling still in your heart. Better still, share the memory. For most of you, life just keeps getting in the way. Take care to not get in your own way. There are no guarantees that you won't at some point in your life get hurt, but life's all about learning, right? Wouldn't you rather be open to the fantastic adventures life has to offer and open your hearts and souls to the beauty all around you?

Mirror Work

When you feel ready to take the next step to self-love, get in front of a mirror and just say "Natasha, I love you", except do use your own name here! When you go up to the mirror and look into your own eyes, you are connecting with yourself, validating yourself, accepting and approving of yourself. The reason most of you feel uncomfortable about trying mirror work is that you have become disconnected with yourself. This is the same reason you avoid eye contact, because you are afraid of the connection to yourself and other human beings. You are here on this earth living in a human body and yet still a spiritual entity, and you came here to connect. So, little by little, learn to accept and then to embrace it.

Once you get into a routine of mirror work, you will find that you accept yourself more, and you may feel more confident. Have fun and be playful with it. Wink at yourself each time you look at a mirror, or tell yourself you look fab. This is to get you to be comfortable with yourself; why wouldn't you want to be? The truth is, most of us are not. We have never really learned to love ourselves. How many times were you told as a child, to not be selfish? To share your sweeties with the other child? The fact is that you are not truly in a position to be able to help another in the real sense of the word, unless you are in a good place yourself.

Mirror work helps you to connect to yourself and with yourself. It helps you form a stronger bond with yourself. When you are forced to come face to face with who you really are, you learn acceptance and non-judgement. Over time, you start to enjoy the connection. You are always there with a welcoming smile to greet yourself. You are not surprised when you see your face, and it feels like home. You notice the judging and the scolding falls by the wayside. Looking in the mirror keeps you grounded. It reminds you of who you are. Mirror work is very powerful in helping you heal. Make mirror work your daily ritual. I do my mirror work each night before I go to bed. It only takes a couple of minutes and is comforting. You can say your affirmations at the same time.

You will learn to rely on yourself in a deeper way, to trust your instincts and to get to know who you are underneath all of the beliefs and guises that society creates. Last thing at night, stand in front of the mirror and tell yourself 8 things that went well for you that day, things you feel proud of. These are just little things such as "Well done for getting the packed lunches made for the kids and taking your wife a cup of tea before you left for work" or "You did a great job at picking up the shopping on your way home." The reason this works so well is that you are congratulating yourself for what went well for you. This is self-care. This is a crucial part of your development and growth. The other reason for adopting this bedtime ritual is that is sets the scene for your sleep. What you are doing in essence is setting up your mind for the 8 hours' sleep you are going to get, with the intention of self-care, positivity and gratitude for how well you did. During the night when your body is resting, your mind gets to work with this. What you focus on comes into view, so your subconscious, which takes up 95% of the mind, can lovingly hold you in a state of joy, harmony and peace.

By comparison, and just to give you an alternative view point, what sort of state do you think the mind is in following a fight with a partner, or watching a violent or frightening movie? Now that you have some insight to the results you are inadvertently giving your mind each and every day, you have the power to change them. When you watch a comedy or have a great evening out with friends, roaring with laughter, this has the same positive effect. Likewise, in the morning, before you even open your eyes, you can say in your head 5 positive outcomes you want for the day. You can even thank your bed for a restful night's sleep or thank the day for giving you a brand new opportunity to achieve amazing things.

Congratulate Yourself

The reason this is important is because many of you are too

tough with yourselves. When you have a child, you encourage them to try walking and say "well done" when they can. You praise them when they finish their food, especially if half of it doesn't end up all over your newly painted wall. You acknowledge achievements both big and small, all throughout their childhood, because you want to encourage success in them and because you love them. So why is it that you forget to do the same for yourself? You see, that's where I find it hard to accept that these techniques shouldn't be mainstream. They should be taught at home, at school and reminded of in the workplace. Why? Because there would be a far smaller number of people with self-esteem issues if everyone were taught this throughout their lives. Yes, okay, you do get the odd "nice one Jack" from your mates, or "that was brilliant darling" from your mother, but by and large it doesn't happen often.

Congratulating yourself is an easy way for you to keep yourself going if it starts to get tough. Your boss might yell at you, your husband might be mad at you, but you can still say to yourself, "Do you know what, you did okay today. You made all the staff laugh with your funny jokes" or "You set yourself a personal goal to complete that report today and you nailed it!" In the same way that a child needs encouragement and we give it without thinking, we all have an inner child that still needs to know they are doing a good job.

So, for this reason, I implore you to take the bull by the horns and get in front of your mirror in the bathroom before you jump into your warm and comfy bed, and congratulate yourself for everything that you have done well today. They don't have to be huge things, like completing a month-long assignment or closing a 3 month deal. They can be the little things that you can say "well done" to yourself about. 10 is a good number, but if that seems too much right now, then start off with 5. I guarantee that before long, once you're in the flow and congratulating yourself each night, you won't want to stop. What you are doing here is acknowledging what went right for you that day. This also sets the intention of sending you to bed feeling good about yourself, so that for the next 8 hours, your mind works with that. Amazing. Do you think you could try that and develop it into a new habit? Now you do need to keep up this habit for more than a couple of days and make it part of your life. Around 60 days should do it. This has the added benefit of clearing your mind of all the other chatter, so you are learning mindfulness at the same time. Do you think you might want some of that? Off you go.

Kindness

To be yourself, to be authentic, to be kind, is to live in alignment with your higher self. Learning to be kind to yourself, others, nature and everything around you elevates you to a position of gratitude and abundance. By showing kindness to others, it opens up your heart and theirs. It is so easy to smile at a stranger waiting for the train, or in a queue. You might end up having a riveting conversation that brightens both your days. It doesn't cost anything to be thoughtful. To hold the door open for the person right behind you could become second nature to you, and will be so much valued. Little gestures such as these make other people feel special and warm inside.

Just imagine, if each and every one of you just smiled at just one more person each day and said "good morning" to someone you have never seen before, offered to hold the lift for someone or help carry a pushchair up some stairs in a shopping mall. The happiness and the feelings of appreciation would spread and, before you know it, everyone you come into contact with during the course of the day would be joyful and relaxed. This would affect your work in a very positive way, and make you more productive. It could have the knock-on effect of cheering up your boss, or getting recognition for your hard work. You would be more likely to be noticed by others around you and in turn congratulated for your efforts and kindness. Gestures of kindness bring smiles to people's faces. A smile is contagious, so is a laugh. This sounds like an imaginary utopia, I hear you say. But actually, it only takes a small gesture of kindness, consideration, or thoughtfulness to lift the mood of everyone around you.

Just think about it for a moment. If you went to bed with positive thoughts in your head, you would sleep more peacefully, feel happier with yourself when you awoke, have a higher self-esteem, have a more enjoyable day at work, feel appreciated by those around you, even if you didn't know them, and at the end of the day you would go home with a spring in your step. You would be much more likely to have a wonderful evening if when you arrived home your mood was lifted. So why is it that, particularly in the western world, we find it so very hard to be happy, positive, thoughtful and kind to one another?

Happiness is a state of mind. It is not something that happens when someone does something for you, or when your ideal partner comes along and sweeps you off your feet and makes you happy. That's very short-lived. No, the responsibility to be happy lies very much on your own shoulders. This is a refreshing concept, don't you think? Because you don't have to rely on anyone else to make you happy. You were born happy; that's just the way it is. Look back far enough and you will remember. It's not you who started off unhappy, it's the prejudices and beliefs you were brought up with, the environmental factors around you and the social pressures and expectations of who you should be, what you should do, what you should have. The "keeping up with the Joneses" madness that you see all around you. Don't get me wrong here, I am not suggesting that you don't go for what you want, or that you shouldn't work hard to achieve what is important to you, or that wanting a 6 bedroom, 5 bathroom detached house with indoor pool overlooking the sea is a bad dream to have. What I am suggesting is that being happy in yourself, rather than looking towards outside influences, is what really counts. In fact, when you combine the needs of the head and the heart with equal passion, you reach your bliss. Striving for success in business is only enhanced by recognising the need for and embracing a heart centred approach. There are many successful people who have achieved this balance, who have uncovered the treasures of the universe and as such live a blissful and complete life, and in turn give back to others and gladly share their secrets. When you act from a point of heart centre, what you desire to see is for everyone around you to become as happy and fulfilled as they can be.

Kindness comes from the heart. It is the act or deed that is offered without anything wished for or expected in return. It is sending out a little piece of love unconditionally to another human being. It is enjoying the look of gratitude on another person's face when you have shown them kindness and the art of giving, not wishing to receive back. It is functioning at the level of bliss, just because you can. Kindness comes from love and love is energy, the most powerful of energies that can make huge changes when harnessed by people at the same time. When you put your intention out there to send love to a place, a person or a nation, when you do this in a group, incredible changes occur. Having the intention is simply stating what you wish to happen as if it has already happened. When you send love to the person you have just had an argument with, even when they do not know, their mood will calm and the tension will disappear. Next time you have a fight with your loved one, try this technique.

Your Takeaway New Daily Exercise

Your takeaway message here is that your daily requirement is 1 hug for survival, 2 hugs for maintenance and 3 hugs for growth. Set that as your new ritual for each and every day. Hug your children, your spouse, a colleague, your very best friend. You can even hug your favourite person twice!

Chapter 2
Acceptance

Accepting Yourself and Others

Acceptance is all about learning to like yourself, just the way you are. Your body, hair, eyes and special unique skills are perfect for you in this lifetime, and were given to you for a reason. It is up to you to accept and learn to love who you are and figure out a way to shine. Learn to love, accept and believe in yourself. Everyone is always doing the best they can with the tools, skills and knowledge they have, at this very moment. By discovering new techniques, such as self-love, acceptance and forgiveness, you can enhance your life. Over time you will accelerate to the next level of consciousness. You will start to understand that you are part of something far greater than yourself. That you are held in the arms of the universe. That you are amazing and perfect just the way you are, and that collectively you are all connected to a higher source or energy. You may think of it as the universe, source, god, or whatever sits comfortably with you. The important point here is to understand that you are all valued the same. You are here to connect, collaborate, co-operate and learn your lessons, have adventures and fun, and enjoy all the wonders that the world has to offer.

By accepting yourself and who you are, you cease the fight and the internal conflict ends. There's no need to judge yourself. You will discover great peace when you come to terms with who you are. By accepting others, there's no need to criticise or try to change them. Accepting who they are and who you are is very liberating, empowering, and leads to you trusting more deeply in your own abilities. You see, when you try to change who you are in any way, you are actually saying to yourself that you are not happy with who you are. It is impossible to run away from yourself. You can to a certain extent change the way you look by the clothes you wear, your hair cut and colour, your fitness regime. These are all ways of enhancing yourself. That's not what I am talking about. Stop thinking you are not good enough. When you completely love and accept who you are, everything works in your life.

You may argue that what I am hinting at is taking away the right of self-expression. That's not the case. Be yourself, absolutely. However, think very carefully about changing your appearance for good, if it is freedom from yourself that you seek. Dig deep and ask the question "Am I happy with who I am?" You are the way you are for a reason. Those who celebrate who they are appear happier, more confident, and shine their light in this world more brightly. Those who accept and enjoy themselves appear to be more at ease in their own skin. That is because they have learned to fully accept who they are, and they are comfortable with themselves . There is always going to be someone younger, taller, slimmer, blonder, and more muscular than you are. Actually, that's fine because we come in different shapes and sizes and no one of us is the same. This also means that each one of us is unique and amazing.

Never be too shy to step into your own magnificence.

Go ahead; get a pen and paper and ask yourself:

1   Who am I ?
2   Why am I here?
3   What are My gifts?
4   How can I share those gifts with the world?

Gratefulness

Focus on what you have that's wonderful in your life, rather than what you don't, and magnificent things will be attracted into your life. By focusing on the good stuff, the universe works to support this and gives you more of the same. When you focus on what's not working for you, or areas that are lacking, you also receive more of the same. So be careful what you focus on and wish for. What you focus on always comes into view.

Being grateful is a way of nurturing yourself; it makes you feel good. What you send out always comes back to you, so when you are grateful for the man who opened the door for you in the pouring rain, or when the woman at the reception desk smiled at you, that makes you feel good. When you appreciate the sunset or the sunrise, when you feel in awe of the clouds, nature and the birds, you fill yourself up with gratitude; it comes back to you and you will get more of the same.

So the next time you get the opportunity to show a little kindness, allow someone else to feel the gratitude for what you did. The only real power you have is in this very moment. So by giving 100% of your attention to this present moment, you can enjoy it all the more. Take the time to really enjoy this moment. You tend to switch off and go into auto pilot when you complete habitual tasks, such as brushing your teeth, doing the washing up or having a shower. You probably do it in exactly the same way as you have always done. If you brush your teeth at the top first, mix it up a bit, and start at the bottom. This will force you to become more mindful of what you're doing and therefore bring you into the present moment. The next time you take a shower, really feel the water washing off all of the negativity of the day, all the regrets you may have had, and those lost opportunities, and let them go. Showers are a very symbolic way of cleansing yourself, so don't miss on the opportunity to clean away all of the sadness, anger or pain. Taking a shower is a very freeing thing to do.

Thank You

Do you always remember to say thank you? Do you thank the bus driver for taking you safely to your destination? Do you thank the shop keeper for serving you? Do you thank the driver who allows you to pull out on the motorway when you are in a hurry? Saying thank you doesn't cost you anything and yet goes a long way. Each time you say thank you, you send positive energy to the other person. Next time you get the chance to say thank you, take it and see how good it feels.

When you are at a family concert or festival and you are far away from the stage, it is the tallest people who have the best view. In order for your children to get a good view, they will need to sit on your shoulders. In life, there are people all around you who have given you a lift up, helped you along the way. Those who have paved the way, in order that you could benefit from their wisdom and continue on that little bit wiser or more in the know. There are those in your life who have been the ones you have stood on the shoulders of. It is so important to recognise that and thank them for enabling you to get the best view. Albert Einstein gave thanks each and every day of his life. He thanked all those amazing scientists and people who stood before him and paved the way for him to go ahead and develop the work he did.

Who do you need to be thankful for? Who is it in your life, in the past or present that you want to thank? There are teachers everywhere you look. What's fantastic is that once you start to become aware and notice those around you who are helping you, everywhere you turn, you will see them. These angels, helpers or just people if you prefer, are there to guide the way for you. They are showing you the direction best for you, teaching you the lessons you need to learn. Next time you go out to work, shopping or for a walk, be mindful of the teachers who may appear before you. Those who are inadvertently there to shine a light for you. Those perhaps in your life already on whose shoulders you stand. They may be your grandparents or other relatives, they may be your friends. Some people come into your life for a very short while, others stay for some time, and the really special ones remain with you forever. Remember to say thank you to them all. See how happy thanking them makes them and you feel.

Remember to say thank you to everyone who helps and serves you in your life. Learn also how to be of service to others. This strengthens the bond between you. Show kindness to everyone you meet. The next time you thank someone, take a moment to really look at them and feel the thanks you are giving. By thanking them, you are blessing them and speaking to them on a much deeper level; you are connecting with their soul. Hold their gaze and see how that makes you feel. See how they respond.

Accepting Change

Accept your situation until such time as you can change it. There is wisdom in this when you look a little closer. There are people all the world over in situations they are unhappy with. You may be unhappy at work, find it difficult growing up in an unloving home, be a victim of emotional or physical violence, or whatever. Nothing lasts forever and so in most cases, you have a choice. You either accept wholeheartedly the situation you are in or you decide to take action to change it. Taking action requires courage. It also means you need to rely on yourself to lead you in the right direction. In the short term, there may be fallout, upset or anger. When you allow yourself to focus on the outcome and intention you desire, you can get through almost anything.

Accepting the change that may occur through no fault or input of your own is more difficult in some respects. When the company you work for is taken over, there lies uncertainty ahead regarding your position. This is a change you will need to accept, or if you cannot, then begin to look for another post. When a family is broken apart as a result of a marital breakup, it's either the apparently innocent partner who was possibly unaware, or certainly the children, who are the innocent bystanders and therefore become the unfortunate victims. The mention I made of the "apparently innocent partner" may have annoyed you and this was not my intention. However, in all relationships, there are signs before the storm. There's always a warning of the wind changing, the coolness and damp feeling in the air, the dark clouds rumbling ahead and the sky turning black. Something within that relationship was going wrong long before the break up occurred. It may have been a mutual growing apart for both adults. It may have been a long, drawn out deterioration that was either never addressed or never properly acknowledged by one party. When you ignore the needs of yourself or another, the problems start to occur.

When you find yourself the victim of an earthquake or flood and all your possessions are lost, the change you need to accept has a high price. Your whole life is turned upside down and the reality kicks in that you have to start over in every area of your life. You would think that anyone would find this devastating, and I am certain that most do. But the strange things is that many people who have experienced such enormous loss in the blink of an eye have found that starting over for them is a liberating experience, one that allows them to rethink everything they once knew. To start their lives over, almost as if they were given a second chance. People, who have experienced such horrendous times have gone on to take a very different path in their lives. Life is a series of lessons that allow us to develop and grow as human beings. To enrich our lives and allow us to not only glimpse the beauty all around, but to wholeheartedly embrace it.

Awareness

Once you become aware that your life is not working for you anymore, or at least not working well, or that there's something missing, then you are ready to explore what is out there waiting for you. The truth is that when you are ready to learn, your teacher will appear. Awareness that some element of your life is not working for you is the first step for you to heal yourself. Once you become conscious of that void, you can look for ways to fill it.

It may be that you look in the mirror one morning and don't recognise the person looking back at you, the person you have become. You might decide that you are not ready to be the sloppy Joe you have become, just yet. You may think that it's about time you started to take care of yourself. You may realise that feeling in your gut each time you go to work, and it may suddenly dawn on you that this feeling is a sign. A sign that your body has been trying to tell you about for months or perhaps even years. When you are ready to listen to your body, you start to notice little things. Your body is giving you messages all the time. When you feel tired, lie down. When you feel anxious, take time to breathe. When you have a gut feeling in your stomach, there's a message there too. If it feels like a knot, then your body is trying to tell you that what you are doing is not in alignment with who you really are.

Awareness comes also with an element of responsibility. You have noticed and now you need to pay attention and maybe even be prepared to take action. As your awareness grows, your intuition will lead you to the answers and guide you. Your mind is incredible and gradually you will become conscious of certain feelings or outcomes that will lead you to the right path. It may be a book someone gives to you, or perhaps a meeting you are invited to attend. Be prepared to take these small steps and follow that inner voice. Your intuition is your inner guidance system that will never lead you into harm's way, but instead hold your hand and take you gently from the shadows into the light if you allow it to.

We were all born with an internal guidance system, our intuition, and most of us were never taught how to use it. It is only when you become curious that you start to seek out more knowledge. Some people remain completely content living the life they have chosen, without any thought for more. Or they might be blissfully happy in their ignorance or fearful of change, and so never push the boundaries of their own personal development. It is only when you become aware and the penny drops, so to speak, that you realise there may be more out there to life. Your journey back to yourself can only start when you have this awareness. It isn't for everyone and that's fine. It is, however, like opening Pandora's Box. Once opened there can be no going back. The treasures that lie before you are too beautiful and cannot be denied. To relish in the amazingness of the universe is too powerful a force on a mortal's soul. After all, the universe and all its glory are there for you to enjoy and experience.

The knowledge and the wisdom you seek is out there for you. All you have to do is be ready and receptive. Listen to the little voice in the back of your head. With awareness comes consciousness, and this leads to awakening. The process of awakening, more often than not, takes time for most people. It is a gradual developing of the senses. You will start to notice small things at first. You might hear sounds you never heard before. You may be aware of the birds singing when you weren't previously listening. It could be the vibrant, delicate flowers in the park or your own garden that catch your eye and take you by surprise. A butterfly, floating in front of you minding its own business, may have a profound effect on you. Your world may appear clearer, brighter, and more colourful. These are all little signs that your energy is changing, that you are waking up to the wonders of the world. It's a truly intoxicating feeling, one which you may find is accompanied by an enormous wave of emotion. You could feel joy in abundance, you may burst out crying. There's nothing wrong with either reaction; it's just that you may never have seen with those eyes before.

Accept The Way You Are

Accept the way you are. You are perfect, amazing and unique just the way you are; it's how you were made. It's no accident you came out this way. There's not another human being quite like you, and that makes you so very special. Have faith in your own abilities and believe in yourself, no matter what. Learn to rely on your own inner wisdom, your intuition, your inner guidance system. Accept the way things are for you, let go and trust. The universe will provide for you. Mother earth holds you in her arms and keeps you safe. You are a child of the universe and have a very important job to do. The only matter you need to concern yourself with is what your skills and gifts are and how best you are to use them. Everything else is just noise.

New Daily Takeaway Rituals – Discover who you are & what your gifts are

Start off with a piece of paper. Go get one now and I will wait for you.

Great! Okay, so now draw two vertical lines down the page from top to bottom, splitting the page into three equal parts.

At the top of the page, on the left hand side, write the heading "Things I Love Doing"

In the centre column, write the words "Things I Am Really Good At"

Then on the right hand of the page in the final column, write the heading "Things I Don't Like"

Now be really honest with yourself when you write these items down.

Add anything and everything that applies here and take no notice of what others might think. Their opinions are none of your concern. This is your life and you won't get a second chance if you make a mistake.

Remember what you are doing is discovering and acknowledging what your skills and gifts are. We all have them, so don't even think about writing nothing. It may be hard at first, but once you think about what you did as a child, or as a teenager that made you laugh or what you tried and were really good at, those are your gifts. You might be an ideas person, so put that down; you could be a fabulous skier. Perhaps you love to bake, but doubt whether it would pay the bills. Hold nothing back; these are your gifts, no one else's. You could ask those around you whom you trust to pinpoint a few for you. Add them to your list.

When you have finished and you are satisfied there's nothing left out, look down the list of "What You Love To Do" and "What You Are Great At".

Highlight all of the words that match in both of these sections and leave the rest. Ponder on the highlighted list, it may be long or short, but it's your list.

There you will find a clue to what you need to be doing in your life to make you happy in your work. There are many people who are doing what their parents expected them to do, what society would approve of or what would pay the most money. These are not the careers you need to pursue; these are not the roads you walk down to happiness. Follow your heart in such matters. Be led by your intuition. Do you suppose Tiger Woods thinks he might be better off as a car mechanic? No, of course not. He has found and embraced his true life's purpose. Have you found yours? I hope this exercise has helped you.

Chapter 3
Forgiveness:
The Ultimate Gift to Yourself

Forgiveness is the fragrance the violet sheds on the heel that has crushed it.
- Mark Twain

Holding Onto Resentment

Resentment is one of the more cruel lessons that you might not learn. I hope that by sharing this with you, you can find it in your heart to take yourself through the steps of forgiveness. Holding onto a wild animal who cuts, bites and hurt us is what it feels like to hold onto resentment. It starts off with arrogance, the thought that you are right and the other person is wrong. Then it turns into stubbornness, digging your heals in, where there is no way you are going to back down from your point of view, as it's a question of principles. You will have heard someone in your life, or even yourself say "It's the principle; I wouldn't have stuck to my guns so much, but really, they absolutely enraged me..." There are feelings of hurt, anger, pride, principles and non-forgiveness here. All these emotions will only bring unhappiness and ill health. When resentment takes hold and you become so stuck in the treacle that you are unable to move, that is the time to take heed.

You see, bottling up how you feel, refusing to budge and standing your ground over a matter that is probably so trivial that over time you have forgot what the argument was all about anyway, doesn't make any sense. Over time, if left unresolved, you begin to internalise your anger and maybe even play out the scene over and over in your head, each time you do so feeling a small sense of justice when you think of the right words to say, in your head. You may even go over and over the same scenario day in and day out for weeks, months or even years. From an outsider's point of view, this might seem like a completely mad thing to do. It may look as if you have stopped living and got caught up in the ropes. Truth is that's exactly what you have done, stopped moving forward. When you become stuck in that resentment, pride, principle, anger cycle it is difficult to see the wood from the trees. The feelings this produces overflow into each and every area of your life and you begin to almost suffocate unless you can find a way to let go.

The next time you find yourself in a situation not dissimilar to this one, my desire is that you become aware of what you are doing. Be aware that this is your life and it's okay. Everyone is different and that's why there are so many varying views. Actually, it's this variety that gives life its rich tapestry. You start to realise the craziness of pride and principles getting in the way. The behaviour that could damage you and others around you. Never mind the energy you are wasting on it. And with a bit of luck you can catch yourself and laugh as the penny drops at what you have been doing. Don't think for a second that you are alone; people do it all the time. The crazy thing is that we have been accepting this as the norm. Why did you never question that this sort of self-talk wasn't helping, and certainly not solving the problem?

The point here that is so important for you to grasp, is that it isn't only you who gets dragged down into the darkness, the pits of resentment, but all those around you. As if it's not bad enough that you allow yourself to suffer by holding onto resentment, to curl up and become literally rigid with this disease. Even your bones will harden, becoming brittle when you are unable to release the feelings that resentment creates. Your family, friends and colleagues will all be affected by the deep rooted poison that is resentment as it seeps out of you through every pore. It eats away at you from the inside and leaves nothing. When you look around you, you will notice people who are set in their ways, stubborn, principled, narrow minded, seldom opening their hearts. Some sadly shut themselves off from the world and no longer flow through life like the river that runs freely.

When you see others who carry this heavy burden, hopefully you will be able to recognise it for what it is and feel sadness in your heart for them. You can bless yourself, and then bless them. Let your awareness also act as a reminder of the necessity to release any negative feelings towards yourself or others. To accept that holding a grudge, proving a point is so utterly pointless. Does it even really matter anyway? What difference does it make in your life, when you do not agree with another person? Do you want to spend so much of your precious time mulling over scenes in your head that no longer serve you?

Your life was not meant to be difficult; it wasn't supposed to be a struggle. Remember that your life was created to be amazing. Find the space in your heart to be open, to feel safe enough to let go of any feelings of resentment and to move slowly into the light that will release you and set you free, and shine from every part of you. Once you understand that all your thoughts create your future, you begin to become more selective about the thoughts you think.

Forgiveness Sets You Free

Now I don't know about you, but when I first came across this particular word, it may as well have been an enormous, hairy, scary monster. You may feel the same as I did; that there was no way that you could bring yourself to forgive this person or that person. But the truth is, if you really want to set yourself free and live an authentic life, then forgiveness is the only way. I'm not suggesting that you just go down that dark and terrifying forgiveness road all by yourself, you will need 2 friends to tag along. Love and acceptance are always happy to help and they will give you the strength to face the people and things you need to forgive.

Now forgiveness isn't just about forgiving the other person, it is also about forgiving yourself. It is a mountain to climb, no doubt. The mountain that indeed needs to be climbed is only made possible by attempting one step at a time. The great news is that this mountain, once climbed, will set you free. In forgiving yourself, you lighten your load. You all carry around far too much mental baggage. At times it feels as though you are dragging around all your possessions with you. The weight of this can feel like a car or a house at times. You begin to feel over time that it's hard to breathe. You feel exhausted. Eventually, your body has had enough and sometimes even stops you in your tracks, by creating illness or dis-ease.

When you choose to forgive another person as well as forgiving yourself, it will set you free. You feel so free, you could almost fly. Forgiving to the point of "as if it has never happened," now that's a biggie; I get that. So if that's a step too far for now, then just forgive the person who wronged you. And also forgive yourself for feeling the way you do. In situations where the person who requires forgiveness is not around anymore, has moved away or no longer contactable, you can still perform this forgiveness on them. All you need to do is begin by closing your eyes. You probably will want to be alone in a quiet place where you feel safe. If you are able to, then imagine they are at the other side of the room. Take a deep breath and imagine you are forgiving them. As you state your intention, visualise them as becoming relieved and see them in your mind's eye as happy. See them as if they truly value this forgiveness you have shown them. They are free and so are you. If you can do this in person, great. If you are brave enough to call or write, then you simply refer to the unkind act or word and state briefly and clearly that you forgive them and that you would like very much for them to in turn forgive you.

If it is you who needs to be forgiven, ask the other person for forgiveness. Try saying something like "Do you remember some time ago I said this and it really hurt you? Then after that we didn't really talk. What I would really like is to ask you to forgive me because it has made me very sad to think that we might not be friends anymore. Would you consider forgiving me so that we can both move on?" Now that doesn't sound too difficult, does it? This is incredibly powerful. In fact, if you're feeling like you couldn't face the other person, you can carry out this same process in the safe, warm environment of your own home. The important point is that you say sorry with feeling and intent. That you truly are sorry in your heart. Then the guilt, shame, and embarrassment will all disappear. It has the power to set you both free, to lighten your load, to stop dragging you down. The journey of life at times seems hard enough without any extra baggage.

Forgiving Yourself

To forgive yourself is to accept who you are. You are the best you that you can be. To stand in your magnificence and just be. Be yourself, as there's no point pretending. To love yourself and everything you are. To see yourself in all your glory, as a spiritual being living in a human body and living a human life. The peace you feel, that emanates from you, when you know who you are. Once you can fully embrace the difference between your essence and your physical being, you can rejoice at the fantastic sides of soul and form. To fully appreciate your senses, the touch of support from a loved one, the smell of a flower in full bloom, the singing of the most amazing opera singer, holding hands for the first time with your soul mate, the gentle, warm, soothing kiss on your child's face, the taste of the spring rain on your tongue. These are the things that will help you be heart centred, so that only love flows in and radiates out. When there's only love, there's no room for resentment or hate.

To forgive yourself is to simply let go. When you can live every day as your true self, the need to hold onto any feelings or emotions that aren't helping you just fades away. To truly let go of everything that doesn't serve you in your life is very liberating. You may need to forgive or let go of the values that don't serve who you are right now. They may have been values in the home when you were a child, values your parents held. When you let go and start to change, everything in your life changes for you and around you. The universe holds you and conspires to help you. You feel supported and provided for. When you focus on what your heart desires and resist the temptation to get caught up in the detail, you no longer wobble, you stride forwards with confidence that you are safe; you see the truth, your path is clear.

When you learn to forgive yourself for everything you have ever forgotten to forgive, it sets you free. . You can practice forgiveness daily in front of a mirror, as an affirmation or part of your breathing technique during a mindfulness moment.

Forgiving Others

As you start to think about the importance of forgiving those who have hurt you, you realise that it is you who will be released from the curse. Many people in your life, who you feel have upset you or caused you harm, won't even be aware of how their actions and words may have affected you. Most people don't deliberately set out to be unkind. Therefore don't be surprised if you tell someone you forgive them and they appear genuinely surprised. Even more reason for you to not hold onto any negative feelings towards them.

These are the powerful lessons of your lives. To practice forgiveness each and every day, to cleanse the soul of feelings, vibes, emotions that do not help in your journey through life. When the marathon runner starts his race, do you see him carrying a huge rucksack on his back? Does he stand at the starting point with bags full of stones? Imagine yourself as that marathon runner. You wouldn't get very far in your life before hitting that proverbial wall, with all the heavy baggage being dragged along, would you?

The steps you can take to sever the ties that bind you in your life and liberate yourself into the most amazing status are easy steps, so long as you stay out of your own way. The road of free thinking, heart centred openness to learning and adopting new ideas, to develop and grow as a human being is paved along the way with the most gorgeous adventures and treasures. These are all for you to enjoy when you take you first step towards a more honest and authentic life. Never, ever again be afraid to stand in your own power, to be proud of who you are and how you can serve others. The journey of your life is the adventure, not the destination. The only power any of us have is in this very moment. Give yourself 100% to this moment, enjoy it, savour it; it will never come again.

When you are required and feel the need to forgive another person, do it with love, either remotely or face to face. It doesn't really matter if you don't feel brave enough to face them. What matters is that you mean it. When you forgive someone for doing wrong unto you, you are setting them free and also you are setting yourself free. When you truly say sorry to another person for what you have said or done to hurt them, this will free you. Bear in mind that you can only change yourself and never another human being, and so be prepared that they may not be ready to forgive you. You can forgive them for that too. When you say the words "sorry" or "I forgive you" your words are more powerful when you say them and feel them too.

Worldwide Forgiveness

Have courage in your heart, allow forgiveness to flow through you like water, trust in who you are and everything that you can be, speak the truth with kindness, serve others, be authentic and follow your intuition that is guiding you safely though your life. Never allow doubt to creep into your mind like a thief in the night, and sabotage what your essence has created. There is no route to happiness; happiness is the way. At all times remain positive, open, flowing, accepting, and throughout it all have love at your core.

Over the millenniums many atrocities have occurred throughout history. Many people have perished, died and been killed due to genocide, wars, religious crusades and so on. It's not enough to forgive another person for hurting you; whole tribes and nations need to be forgiven too. It is the responsibility of us all, to act from a point of acceptance. We all breathe the same air, come into the world and leave this planet in the same way, comfort one another when times are hard, and have the need to connect and communicate. The entire world over has babies who need their mother's love. We all need shelter, food, water and warmth. We are not so different, wherever we live.

You each have it in your hearts to forgive. Love is the most powerful energy force that exists, and if only half a community set the intention to send love and peace to the other half of the community, there would be peace in the whole community. It is not the fault of the children, grandchildren or great grandchildren to be held accountable for the terrible acts of violence of their forefathers; that's nonsense. It is up to each and every one of us to forgive the past and live in the present, in an accepting and loving way. War only brings more war, hate only brings more hate, resentment only brings more resentment. But love only brings more love, understanding and collaboration. Where love stands, there can be no hate.

The only way to have peace the world over is through love. When each one of us makes the choice to change, everything changes. In a place where there is no love, you must bring love. These are your lessons. When you put love out there, when you begin to live your truth, people will come into your life to help you along your journey. The whole world shifts to become aligned with your true purpose. When you respect another human being, when you completely accept them for who they are, when judgement is no longer present, when love is in your heart, that's when the world will forgive.

"Forgiveness is the fragrance the violet sheds on the sole of the shoe that crushes it."

New Daily Take Away Rituals

I have handpicked this ritual for you to practice that complements perfectly your forgiveness of others. Forgiveness was one of the hardest things to do in my own life and this is how I managed to forgive others.

Take yourself somewhere quiet where you won't be disturbed. When I did this I went to my bedroom and sat on the bed, but you can sit anywhere you feel comfortable.

Close your eyes and take a few deep and measured breaths.

Imagine that in front of you is a stage.

On the stage, visualise a person in your life who you really need to forgive.

They may be living or not.

Picture this person sitting on a chair in the middle of the stage. Know you are safe as they are a long way from you.

Imagine that you are smiling at this person and wishing them a happy life. You wish them peace in their heart.

As you look at them, you notice that they also smile back, as if they understand what you are thinking.

Be mindful to not bring any judgement to the situation, just peacefully wish them well.

Once you can feel peace in your heart, you can imagine the person just disappearing.

If you find this difficult, as I did, then choose another person to begin with.

All the people who have ever said or done anything to hurt you in any way will need forgiving, including yourself if you have hurt someone else.

By following these guidelines, you are releasing those who have been unjust to you and at the same time, you are setting yourself free.

When you hold onto any type of resentment for whatever reason, it acts as a heavy weight around your neck and that is why you need to let go.

It is you who you are setting free, by forgiving them.

The ultimate in forgiveness is to reach the point where you decide that the thing you are forgiving never even happened. Now that's a deep form of forgiveness and one that may take time to master.

Don't carry around unnecessary burdens as they will weigh you down.

Chapter 4
Stop Worrying, Stop Criticising, Excuses Be Gone

It is, I feel, my duty to impart to you the message that your life is for living. To guide and inspire you to open your heart and follow your heart's desire.

Fear

Babies are born with no fear.
No fear of falling
No fear of failing
No fear of hurting
No fear of asking for exactly what they want – food, drink, love, sleep.
Then we systematically teach them fear!
Don't do this because you'll fall over and hurt yourself.
Don't go too close to the fire because you will get burned.
Don't go too close to the water's edge because you will fall in.
Don't throw your food, you'll make a mess.
Don't put your hands in your food, you'll make then dirty.
Then we justify the need to have FEAR and instil it in our children under the guise of keeping them safe.
Don't talk to strangers, they can't be trusted.
Don't walk into the road, you'll get run over.
Don't go out on your own, it's dangerous.
And so on, and so on, and so on.
Do you recognise this pattern?

Once this fear that our parents created in us, thinking they were helping, has become entrenched in our psyche it's there to stay. Before long it has taken hold and become second nature and starts to control us. This fear holds us back and stops us from living a full life.

Don't buy that car, you can't afford it.
Don't buy that house, the mortgage will cripple you.
Don't bother talking to that girl, she's way too good for you.
Don't set your sights on him, he's successful, rich and famous and out of your league; or whatever.

We restrict our lives, put ourselves in boxes that hold us tight, restrict our creativity coming alive, and prevent ourselves from breathing. We make our world a little smaller.

What holds you back? Fear. What are you afraid of? Fear of failure, fear of rejection, fear of standing out, fear of being different, fear of success. When fear gets in the way of you achieving what you want in your lives, some of you stop. Don't give up. Find a way around that barrier. Make a decision that what you want is greater than the obstacle in your way. Then with this desire to overcome what stands in your way, you will find a solution to solve this challenge and get there. When you give more, when you try harder, when you put yourself out, that's when life gives you more back.

How can you open your heart to the possibilities ahead of you when you are filled with fear? Fear holds you back from your own brilliance. Get out of your own way. Stand fast, stand in your own power and be prepared to own it. Move forward from a place of fear to one of unfolding your uniqueness and become fulfilled. When you begin to move out of your comfort zone, you inadvertently start to conquer your fears. When you confront your fears, embrace the absurd, your brain sets to figure the problems out. Your brain has an amazing capacity to problem-solve, you just very rarely use it. Once you have faced a fear, it seems less scary. When you are in an unpleasant or difficult situation, quietly say to yourself "I choose peace, rather than this."

Open your heart; learn to live a true and full life. You don't want to spend months or even years unlearning the fear that binds you. This is all part of the learning process. It is through the biggest challenges in your life that you learn the greatest lessons. Out of adversity comes opportunity. Out of the chaos comes creativity. Out of fear comes strength. Once you have faced fear and survived it, the next time you encounter the same fear, you are ready. You will have learned how to handle it, your confidence will have grown, and you will be strong and evolved in order to handle it.

You are all creators of your own world. Fear gets in the way and so you forget your creative side. When you choose to live from the point of heart centre and make the decision to be happy, when you can let go and trust, this is when you can step into your power, release the fear and the chains that have held you stuck for so long. Once you learn to rely on yourself, to trust your own judgement and follow your intuition, to really understand that you are safe and that the universe is holding you and supporting you, then and only then can you be set free from the fear that holds you.

You may be scared of revealing your true identity to the world. There is no shame in showing yourself and your vulnerability to the world; this shows great courage and strength. When you remove the mask that you have hidden behind, the one that you feel is acceptable to society, you can be who you really are. For whatever reason, and there are many, so few of you feel able to truly be yourselves. You dress and speak in a certain way because it's how you think others want to see you. You don't feel as though your true colours will be accepted. And yet, when you are not being yourself, the only person you are kidding is you. Be authentic; bring all of you to your business and each area of your life. With love in your heart, be honest and true to yourself and others. Allow your radiance to shine through. You won't lose your power when you are being yourself. And in any case, everyone else is taken! So be the best you that you can be every day.

Beliefs were formed in your mind when you were a child by the values and belief system your parents had. What was acceptable in society or what you were taught through education all have a profound effect on how you value yourself. These beliefs place you in a box, pigeon hole you and then continue to restrict and control you throughout the rest of your life, unless you question, challenge and change those beliefs when they cease to serve you. Your beliefs hold you back, preventing you from living the life of your dreams. It is fear that gets in the way, in all its guises. By changing your beliefs, dropping those that no longer serve you, your decisions will change, your actions will change and before you know it, the results you were getting that weren't working for you will also start to change. Your life will ultimately feel more like it's your life, because you are now living in a way that suits you, that aligns with your purpose.

When you judge or criticise yourself, you stop growing as an individual. When you berate yourself, you hold yourself back. Rather than judge yourself for what you did not achieve today, instead congratulate yourself for all that was good. There are always plenty of things you won't get done; however, as soon as you begin to look, you will find that there is so much that is amazing that you did achieve. Let that be your focus and see how it makes you feel. It's okay to be imperfect. Give yourself permission to not be perfect and embrace that. Step into the highest version of yourself that you can muster. You will expand and grow.

It important to create space, in your mind, to unclutter. Once you begin to allow for space to enter your life, in the form of focusing on the now and becoming present to this very moment, you will be able to watch as your heart starts to open to make way for what it is that you truly desire. The space you create can then allow those desires, wishes and dreams to come into your life in ways you never expected. Beware that, when they do, you should embrace them for what they are and be thankful and grateful for receiving them. For if you are not grateful and do not appreciate what you have received, what the universe has just provided you with, you will lose the very thing you set your heart on.

Stop Worrying About Yesterday

Stop Worrying. It's such a waste of your precious energy. All you actually have is right here, right now. Don't give up your power by becoming preoccupied by yesterday. Focus your full attention, without distraction, on what you are doing. Give the present moment 100% of your attention.

Yesterday has gone, it no longer serves you. So why is it that even though you know this to be true, you continue to worry about the past? There may be parts of your past that sadden you, that you regret and that hinder your future. In order to move forward, you need to let go. The past only drags you down. It served you then, but not now. The present moment serves you now. When you live in the past, you get clogged up, you feel like you are walking through honey and it becomes very difficult to move forward.

There will be things for everyone from the past that are debilitating and scary even. However, what do you think happens when you constantly go over and over them in your head? You get stuck, you cannot move. The past may drag you down, feel like a burden and even make you ill. Once you learn to heal yourself, through forgiveness, acceptance and non-judgement, you will be able to move forward with ease. Most of you worry about the same things every day. It becomes a vicious circle. When you consider how busy your lives are with work, families, social pressures and social media making demands on you, it is no surprise you find yourself in the cycle of worry. However, in order for you to move forward, you need to create the space for your brain to find a solution that will work for you in any given situation.

Through practising not worrying any more, you will find that your mind becomes more creative. The time you used to take up with the worries you had can be better used to focus on the now. Your whole outlook will improve when you leave behind the worries.

Now here's the thing. You can't change yesterday and yet you worry about all or your yesterdays in all of your todays. Release any attachment to yesterday that you may be holding onto. Okay, so I fully understand that for you, if your yesterday was particularly painful, letting go will take a good long time. Of course. That's alright, it makes total sense. All pain takes its time to heal. However, for most of you, the things you worry about from your yesterdays are mostly things that you certainly cannot change. So you spend all of your time going round in circles, having the same conversations to yourself in your head, and really when you step back and look at this behaviour, it doesn't make any sense. Whilst you are so busy worrying about your tomorrows, you are missing your todays. Are you with me now?

Stop Worrying About Tomorrow

The past and the future are actually out of your control. So any attempts to try and control them are futile. Why worry about what has not yet occurred? You see, when you use your precious energy and put it into worrying about tomorrow, it won't change the outcome. In fact if anything your worrying will only add to the pressures you put on yourself to achieve perfection each day. It is better, then, to allow tomorrow to take care of itself. The worry about what hasn't happened and what is only imagined is, more often than not, much more severe than the reality when it arrives anyway. So decide you will stop worrying about tomorrow and see the sense in that advice. Once you let go of the whole worrying saga, you will notice a feeling of liberation come over you. You no longer hold onto some imagined scenario in your mind of what might be, but instead trust that everything will work out for the highest good and then let go and trust.

When things go wrong, as they sometimes do, you will need to be alert, aware and ready to take action if necessary. When a real problem occurs, you can breathe and rise above it, metaphorically speaking. As the problem arises, imagine you are hovering above this challenge before you and look down on it to give it perspective. Tell yourself what you see. What you have done here is become objective about what it is that requires your attention, without becoming overwhelmed by the enormity of it. Any action that you may need to take will appear to you more clearly, once you have put some space between it and you. Until that point, you can spend your time and energy on your life at this very moment in time. Use the time wisely and invest your energy in doing what you have more control over.

There's a whole bunch of you who insist on worrying about tomorrow. Now why is that, when tomorrow hasn't even arrived and it will take care of itself in its own good time? When the penny finally dropped for me, it hit me like a bullet. How crazy, to waste all of our todays, when that's all we have, by worrying about all of our yesterdays and all of our tomorrows? Sounds a bit like madness to me.

By giving all your attention to this present moment, you are maximising it. And when you completely focus on what you are doing, the chatter and worry in your head subsides. Remember by focusing on what you want, what you focus on comes into view. In other words, when your focus is on good things, they come into view; when you focus and worry about bad things, that's also what you will find. Are you going to be the one who gives away all your power and allows your thoughts to run your life? Or would you rather take charge of your mind and keep it under control? I will show you how to do this a little later in easy to follow ways.

Stop Criticising Yourself

Learn to honour who you are; don't be nervous about discovering yourself. Be gentle with yourself; learn to forgive everyone, including you. Making mistakes is part of the learning process of being human. When you criticise yourself, you are harming you; when you criticise others, you are harming them and you. We are all connected and so the cycle of pain just continues. Once you come to see this you won't want to criticise anymore. It seems that everywhere you go, you can hear people criticise each other or themselves, or a situation that hasn't worked out for the best for them.

When you are kind to others and yourself, your world expands, and the love that comes from this kindness is shared amongst us all. If you believe, as I do, that where you place your focus becomes visible, and where you place your thoughts and words delivers what you ask for, you may want to choose your thoughts and words more carefully. What you ask for is attracted back to you. You are a magnet. When you ask for good things to happen, when you put the intention out there for amazing things to come into your life, they do. When you focus on your glass always being half empty, that's what you find. When you complain you have no money, that will be your experience. When you feel that everyone who lives in your hometown is unfriendly, wherever you live that's what you will find.

On the flipside, if you find that everyone you meet is friendly and kind and thoughtful, then wherever you choose to live, that will also be your experience. What you look for, you will find. Be compassionate towards others and see how they respond. When you change, everything changes around you, so when you can learn to put worry and criticism behind you, the world will open up to you in ways you have never imagined.

Stop Criticising and Complaining About Others

The culture you live in seems to encourage the criticism of others. It seems acceptable to criticise yourself. Everywhere you go, in a shop, on the bus, at work, even at a party, people criticise and judge. This seems to me a very strange pastime. There doesn't seem to be any point to it, other than to join in with what other people are saying. Criticising never achieves anything positive; instead it creates distance between people. Make a stand and stop following the crowd. Show kindness to others around you, wherever you meet them. When you think of someone you love, your blood pressure drops, your blood vessels expand and your heart opens. On the contrary, when you feel negative or angry, your blood vessels contract and your blood pressure rises. So these very physical signs are directly connected to how you feel. That being the case, you may decide that criticising others no longer holds value for you. Use love instead, and focus your blessings. Each and every day, bless yourself then bless someone else. When you want to make things good between you and another person say "I'm sorry, I love you. Please can you find it in your heart to forgive me? Thank you."

Have you ever noticed how the health of a person who seems to spend a lot of time complaining is? Being miserable, complaining and not laughing and being joyous, sucks the very life out of you. Those who are miserable feel unsupported, and their health eventually suffers. Usually the problems occur in the back, which represents the support system, or the blood, which represents the flow of life, or the heart, where the ability to love and be loved resides. Love and laughter are both very healing, and it is never too late to recognise where you may have been going wrong and take steps to change it.

When a negative thought about someone enters your head, get another one, a positive one. Turn it around each time you start to feel a criticism enter your head. All you need to do is unwrite the programme that created this negative mindset and replace it with a different programme. By repeating a new habit each day, it becomes second nature. The thoughts you think become your reality, so think wisely. When others complain it's unpleasant to listen to. It's worth remembering that complaining and criticising are affirmations. They are negative affirmations. When you put out a negative affirmation, the universe delivers more of the same. When you put out a positive affirmation the universe answers. So the next time you catch yourself complaining, realise that these thoughts and affirmations are not helping you in any way. As they are just thoughts, they can be changed, so change them for thoughts that serve you.

Excuses Be Gone

Have you ever just sat there and listened to someone who is an excuses person? They may be young, middle aged or old. The story, regardless of age, is exactly the same. It goes something like "I couldn't go away this year as I couldn't afford it" or "I wasn't able to get on the housing ladder because I didn't have the deposit" or "I couldn't come to your party because I had too much on." These are the people who, as a result of not stepping out of their comfort zone, hold themselves back. They then love to justify why they couldn't do this or they couldn't do that, with the excuses they tell themselves and others. At the end of a person's life, it is the things they have not done that they regret, not the things they have done. So why is it that, when you are very much alive, you choose to deny your heart's desire and seek refuge in the excuses you give?

Believe it or not, when you enter this world, you have all the tools required to do or achieve anything that you want. It is up to you to discover what you want, what your skills are and how to use them. Ask yourself, "What is it that's important to me?" Be clear about what you want. Recognise what may be holding you back. Look at ways you might be able to eliminate those obstacles. Make space in your life for anything new to come along. You might need to declutter in the process. Give your home and office a spring clean, to make way for new opportunities to come into your life. Set a date for when you want to have achieved them by. These steps will help you get focused on having an action plan that you can implement and follow. Be aware that, in most cases, your environment will conquer your will power and, unless you remain disciplined, you could revert to type.

By giving all your attention to this present moment, you are maximising it. And when you completely focus on what you are doing, the chatter and worry in your head subsides. Whether you focus on good or bad, that's what you will find. If you don't believe me, and I expect at first you won't, then try it. Carry out your own research; spend a week smiling at everyone you pass by. Make a point of saying "good morning" to everyone you meet. Thank people in your email, at the train station, at the coffee shop and truly mean it. I challenge you to have a happier day.

That's my deepest wish for you all, everywhere. Just think what we could be capable of if we all just pulled together and worked in harmony. There are those of you who may feel cross at what I am suggesting and I get it; so did I. You might think that the thoughts in your head have absolutely nothing to do with your body getting sick. But of course they do; body and mind are connected. What if you were told that each time you watch something violent on the television, your body actually feels the same as if you actually witnessed that event? Every time you see the news portraying the atrocities around the globe, it isn't an accident what you are feeling; deep down inside the hurt is so much, almost as if that was happening to your loved ones. This is because firstly we are all connected and when one of you hurts, as a society, we all hurt. It is also incredibly painful because your mind cannot distinguish between an actual experience, a dream, a film you may be watching, or a book you have just finished reading. Are you going to be the one who gives away all your power and allows your negative thoughts to run your life? Or would you rather take charge of your mind and keep it under control? I will show you how to do this a little later in easy to follow ways.

Positive Outcome

When you start to conquer your fears, stop judging and criticising yourself and allow yourself you become challenged by the things that help you grow, you begin to expand. You will feel courage, learn to rely on yourself, and be in a position to be able to give back to the world and help serve others. Ultimately you will make a difference in this world with all of your skills and all of your knowledge. When you decide to bring love to a situation as a way of dissolving a problem, that's enriching. Learn to focus on your own life, rather than trying to change the lives of others. Be ready to offer support; inspire and listen to those around you without judgement.

Adopt an attitude of harmony in your life at home and at work. Use both of your ears to listen to others so that you allow them to speak more than you do. When you do this, others will remember and really feel like you have taken the time with them.

It is my wish for you to feel empowered by the contents of this book. For you to really want to take full and complete responsibility for your life, by achieving personal joy, peace, love and happiness.

New Daily Rituals

Remind yourself that worrying is not going to achieve anything; criticism will eat away at you. Stop doing what you don't love, do what fills up your heart.

Here's a good business practice:

Get a piece of paper and at the top, write the title "All The Tasks In My Business"

Then, two thirds across to the right hand side of the page draw a virtual line, splitting the page in two.

On the left hand side of the page, vertically list all the day to day tasks, even the little ones, and including some you may not currently do yourself in your business.

For those of you who are mainly at home, list all the tasks you carry out whilst at home, even the small ones.

Even when you think you have exhausted your list, you can always add more later as the list is vertical.

Now, on the right hand side of the page, write a number beside each task.

Use the scale 0-10

0 = being an item you really dislike and 10 = a task you absolutely love to do.

When you have finished this exercise, everything without exception that is below an 8, drop from what you do and either discard this totally from your business, or delegate that task to someone else, preferably someone who can do it justice.

Chapter 5
Affirmations & Thoughts

What Are Affirmations?

Affirmations are thoughts and words that are said to yourself on a regular basis. They are positive thoughts and words to help you improve your life. The reason that affirmations are so useful is that they can stop the chatter that goes on in your head all the time. They quieten the noise that torments so many of you with incessant conversation. And in most cases these are the same conversations that you had yesterday and, more than likely, they will be the same conversations that you will have tomorrow. This chatter goes around and around in your head. It doesn't actually go anywhere or achieve anything. What a waste of head space. But when you get that occasional point of clarity that creates a small space in between the thoughts, it feels amazing. It's exhilarating. Your thoughts change your life. So, by that reckoning, you may like to choose your thoughts and words more carefully in the future. Remember that your thoughts of yesterday create all your futures. Be careful what you wish for.

The point here is to alter the habits you are all governed by in your everyday lives. There are many habits that you follow. They are carried out on auto pilot. So things like brushing your teeth, getting dressed, showering, eating your breakfast. In fact with most of these habits, you just go ahead and do them without any thought at all. There are also many habits that you have adopted over the years that are not in the slightest bit helpful in your life, as we have seen earlier in this book. Habits such as worrying, criticising, having conversations in your head that lead to nowhere, and so on.

Once you reach the stage where you catch yourself doing or saying or thinking something that is unhelpful, you can recognise this and take the appropriate action to alter it. Each time a negative thought comes into your head, you can change it. You may look outside in the morning, for example, and notice that it's raining. Your first thought might be "Oh what a horrible day, I'm going to get soaked on the way to work." So to turn this around into a more positive thought or feeling, you might decide to think "Okay, it's raining. The plants haven't had any water for weeks. They need a good drink. I must remember to pack my umbrella for work."

You see, with just a slight change to your thought, you are making it more acceptable and positive rather than a negative thought. Rather than thinking to yourself "I must hurry up, I can't be late. That would be dreadful and I'll be late for the board meeting, and I will arrive all hot and bothered" thus putting lots of pressure on yourself. So instead you could choose "I wonder if I'll be on time today. There's a board meeting and I would rather have the time to relax when I arrive. I wonder if I will get an extra few minutes before the meeting starts." The only difference here is that you have taken the pressure off and turned it into a maybe situation. By just slightly altering your focus, you have given yourself the space required for you to feel more relaxed. You have reached a point of acceptance in a way that, whatever the outcome, it's okay.

Affirmations can be used to turn the negatives into positives at any time. For those of you who worry all the time about what might happen, affirmations and changing your thoughts are really helpful. You can give yourself permission to have a different outcome. And actually any imagined outcome to any given situation is possible. Think of it like a series of roads all over the place. You reach a crossroads; where do you go? Straight on, left or right? You arrive at a roundabout; which turning will you take? You come to a T-junction; left or right? Or do you want to turn around and go back the way you came? You can change your destiny at the flick of a thought. Do I go to dinner with friends or to that party with my sister? Every decision you make will take you to a different future. Once you become more in tune with your intuition, you can listen for the signs that will lead you to the place you most want to go. You start to trust in yourself more and find that you start to get the answers in very subtle ways. Your intuition only ever leads you on the right path, never into danger.

Affirmations can also help you motivate yourself. When I run in the early morning and am on the home run, I have a hill to climb, so most of the time I need my affirmation of "Come on girl, you can do it. You are strong, your legs are amazing, and you are almost there" to help me reach the summit in one piece. A lovely and gentle first affirmation to use is "I love and approve of myself." This is a reconnection to self, an affirmation that allows you to learn to love and approve of yourself. It may seem to you that you would never need to say this because of course you love and approve of yourself. But you would be surprised at how many people really have difficulty with this one. The thing is, this is the foundation and the first to support the building blocks of strengthening yourself, to raise your vibration and to connect with yourself at a much higher level. To connect you with the universe and all of nature.

When you add a positive emotion or feeling to your affirmations it gives them turbo powers. The kind of feelings and emotions that I am talking about here are:

- Love
- Joy
- Peace
- Desire
- Passion
- Kindness
- Harmony

These are all feelings that come from a place of love. Love is the most powerful of all energies. It can bring down walls, governments, and heal nations. It can heal the sick and it can travel miles to a loved one and touch their heart.

Making Affirmations A Daily Habit

Once you adopt affirmations as a daily ritual, you will start to see the benefits in your life. The best way to start is to simply think of 5-10 areas of your life that are important to you, and that you would like to improve. In the form of gratitude you can say to yourself, or out loud, if you are alone "I am strong", "I am peace", "I am safe and secure", "I am successful", "I am well" or anything that you want to improve for yourself. You can also use gratitude by stating each day all the things you are grateful for. It will take you around five minutes to reel off 10 things you want to be thankful for. By simply bringing to your attention the things that work for you in your life rather than those that don't, you will automatically have a better day. So "Thank you for the beautiful blue sky" would work quite nicely. You may normally be in such a hurry to rush out of the house on the morning in a bid to get to work before your boss, that you don't actually take the time to look at the abundance of beauty all around you.

Once you take a moment to look up and see the trees swishing in the morning breeze, or the sheep and cows dotted around the fields, or to listen to the birds' morning chorus, you will begin to appreciate the amazingness of everything that's around you. Making affirmations a daily habit requires a little discipline, sure, but once you have been practising it for a couple of months, then it too will become a habit just like all the rest you have built up along the walk of your life. The easiest way to maintain this is to have a notebook or journal by your bed, on a table where you can scribble down 10 things you are grateful for each day. Once you have exhausted your supply, you can focus on the ones that are really important to you, like your relationship at home or maybe one at work that needs a little more attention to help it be nurtured.

Using Affirmations As Intentions

To set an intention is kind of like making a wish. You state what your heart desires, you imagine that object of desire, say a new car, in detail, then let go. To be specific, you visualise the car of your dreams. You focus on the colour, the interior, any additional features that you have been wishing for, then you feel the biggest feeling that you can, the same feeling that you would feel whilst sitting in this very car. Then you imagine that you already have this car. It is yours. It is parked on your drive at the front of your house. You are standing there waiting to open the door. Your wife or husband or kids are waving at you from your house. It feels so real that you already have this car, that it would be quite difficult for you not to get it. Trust me, if you dare and try this for yourself. You can only put the intention out there for something good, something that your heart desires. Focus on the feeling to own such a car would give you. Then you have to take a huge leap of faith and believe that you already have it, and let go. You have already put your order in; it doesn't need to be done again.

How Powerful Thoughts Are

The mind is an amazing and powerful entity. However, you must learn to use it wisely. Your mind cannot distinguish between reality or memory and the dreams and thoughts you create. The films you watch, the news you see, and the newspapers you read also affect you. When you listen to a disturbing piece of news, when you watch a violent film, your body processes this and stores it up in your mind, as if you were already there. In time, your body reacts to such experiences, especially when you get into the whole experience. It is, of course, escapism. You buy into the fact that anything is possible. By the same token, just as in reality, you know the subject matter of the film is way out, but whilst you are engrossed watching it, you totally buy into the concept and believe it for a while. Bearing this in mind, you may want to think twice before allowing your children to watch films that are not age-appropriate. You might want to consider what you are filling your head with, unless you are able to watch such programmes without attaching emotion to the story.

So why is it that you find it so difficult to accept that you are made up of energy, that you are a spiritual being living in a human body, and that your life on earth is meant to be an exciting, happy and wondrous adventure? That you are a very powerful being, who through the laws of attraction is capable of attracting anything you want into your life. You look at other people and say "Well, he has everything and he's wealthy, has a beautiful wife and fantastic life, but he's just lucky; that would never happen to me!"

So yes, you are totally right; when you think you can't, you are probably right. However, when you think you can, you are also right. Simply by changing your perspective on what you believe for yourself, you begin to shift and start to uncover the incredible treasures of the universe. And the brilliant thing is that there's plenty for everyone. Just because one person is successful or blissfully happy, it's not at the expense of someone else drawing the short straw.

To make this happen for yourself, you can't stand still. You are required to take action. The first thing that needs to change is you. If you continue to do what you have always done and expect the results to change, they won't. You need to take the lead, change your perspective and then gradually, what comes into your life will also change. You may start to find that as your own energies change, the people who are attracted into your life also change. Some people will start to show up in your life, whilst others may fade into the shadows. At first this feels strange. In time, when you feel comfortable with your energy changing, you may want to put the intention out there each time you are in a meeting, a party, a conference, to only connect with those who are like-minded, positive, or who may be able to collaborate with you. The results are astounding.

Once you understand that everything you think, say, feel and hear affects you and creates your future, you become more mindful of the words you use and the thoughts in your head. When you give power and acceleration to a negative thought, and you have and do many times each day, you are creating an environment for unhappiness to come into your life. On the other hand, and this is where the magic starts to unfold, when you create, think and run with a positive thought and really feel that thought inside of you, you start to attract positive things into your life. Imagine where this could take you. Are you feeling excited by this? Do you get that it's empowering? You should be excited, because you are an amazing and unique being, with fabulous gifts to share with the world.

Who do you want to be? What do you want your life to look like? Are your thoughts helping you get there or hindering you? Who is the one person that can change this? YOU. So now that you have some understanding of your power, be careful what you wish for; be mindful of your thoughts as they create your future. Your thoughts of yesterday create your tomorrows. If you are not happy with what you have created so far, then simply change your perspective and change those thoughts. You are in charge of your own destiny, that's for sure.

Your mind is a strong muscle that requires training and discipline. Once you harness the energy and focus your mind on the direction you want to go, feel how you really want to feel with all of the love you can, by imagining your new reality as if you were already living it. By adding feeling or emotion to a thought, you give it supersonic fuel. Bring joy into your own life as well as into the lives of others.

It's worth remembering that you have around 60,000 thoughts every day. Most of these thoughts, up to 90%, are actually the same thoughts that you thought yesterday. With that in mind, start to consciously be aware of the thoughts that pop into your head. If they are the same as yesterday, act on them. If they are negative, change them. If they are dark, you can acknowledge them; imagine they are like black clouds in the sky and without engaging with these negative thoughts, without giving them any power, simply stand back and watch as they float innocuously by. You can take comfort in the fact that a big, black cloud never hovers over your head forever. This too will pass.

You can ask yourself one question with every thought that enters your mind. You can ask, is it useful or helpful? Is this thought advancing me in the direction I want to go, or is it holding me back? If the thought is helpful, keep it. If the thought is damaging to who you are and where you wish to head, leave it behind and move on. Become more disciplined; keep your mind in check. Replace those negative thoughts with positive ones. Focus on what you want; that's what you will bring into view in your life, and that's what successful people do. They don't get caught up with the negative stuff. They don't get sidetracked with what they can't do, they say "next" and move on!

A Poem by Audrey Young, songwriter, singer, poet

Be blessed my brothers and sisters today
I have this to say
Live life today to the full
Be strong like a bull
Today is new
Filled with positive dew
Do whatever you do
Give it your Best Shot
No cutting corners
Doing your Best
And you will pass the Test

Life is so short
But you never should abort
When the problems are high
Just look to the sky
Believe whatever you want to
We all have a kind streak
Today I feel blessed
That I hope you receive
Some of it from me through this poem
I am sending to you
Audrey

Use Affirmations To Heal

As you have seen, affirmations are positive or helpful thoughts and words that can be used to change your focus from a negative to a positive. Over time, you will see how they can block the negative voices in your head for a short while. This gives relief and a sense of security and safety. The more you practice, the more you realise it helps. Using affirmations, and all of the other methods we have talked about, raises your vibration and leads you to a place of peace and tranquillity. The energy inside of you will become more in tune with the energy in the rest of the universe. You will start to notice how other people criticise and worry and maybe on occasion how you do too. The fact that you now notice these things will give you the opportunity to change the way you think and look at the world. You might notice that you feel offended by other people's criticisms or worries and therefore do not wish to follow the crowd any more. You begin to see how that is unable to help you and it may be the motivating factor, the call to action for you to make the changes in your life that you want to see.

Once you make affirmations part of your daily life, you can use them as intentions towards someone who is sick or someone you have fought with and want to send love to. To send a healing affirmation to yourself, you just put your hand gently over the part of your body that ails you and say to yourself, "Every hand that touches my knee is a healing hand" or wherever you are feeling pain or discomfort. When you do this in line with your positive thoughts, good sleep and a healthy diet, and detox your body, you will see changes in your life that will excite you. They come slowly over time. You are in fact going through a transformation of sorts.

You can use the words in an affirmation in silence to calm a troubled child. You can repeat affirmations in your head towards someone you want to send love to. You can say just about anything that you like that resonates with you. Keep your own affirmation notebook. The affirmations used to improve your life and the affirmations for healing will be slightly different, and unique to each of you. So after a heavy session on the squash court, you may need some extra assistance with a painful arm. When you place your hand over the pain and state with belief, "Every hand that touches my arm is a healing one," over time, you will trust in the powers that your body has. It's not a quick fix and you will need to carry out this process many times.

Manifesting

When you manifest something into your life, it is not appearing out of thin air, or being pulled out of a hat. No, on the contrary, it was already there. The difference is that you were not able to see it or believe it, and were therefore unable to manifest it into your life. The concept of manifesting is that of attracting something that you want into your life. In order for you to make this happen, you will need to be very specific about what it is that you want. What colour, shape, smell, size, etc. So if it's an evening dress, you will need to visualise it in all its glory. Hold nothing back and let your imagination run wild. Hold the picture of it in your mind. Add yourself in the image wearing the dress. Picture how your hair will be, what shoes you will wear, what type of jewellery you will have, and so on. Keep it clear in your mind, then trust and let it go. You have, so to speak, put in your request. In addition to this very specific visualisation of manifesting, you need to add in the emotion this new dress conjures up for you. Feel it with all your heart and soul. You may need to speak with a partner, parent or bank manager regarding the cost. You may be required to take action yourself as well as just showing up. So possibly you might put in a few extra shifts at work. What you are doing here is putting it out there, that this is what your heart desires. Then you are putting in place a series of events to aid that occurring. Then you let go and trust. Your manifestations will appear at the perfect time. Sometimes and often when you least expect them.

Vision boards

These are a great way to have fun and keep your focus on what is important to you in your life. The vision board will ward against complacency and act as frequent reminder of what you wanted all those months and sometimes years ago. It is so easy to allow life to wash over you, to sweep you out to sea along with the millions of other people who weren't able to hold onto their dreams. Or who didn't have the courage to dream as big as they would have liked to. Or who were just too scared of failure to even give themselves permission to have a dream.

Well, here's the good news. It's never, ever, ever too late to have a dream. Think it up, dream it big, as big as you can, believe you can have it and then, each and every day, take a small step to get you there. It takes the same amount of energy to dream a little dream as it does a big dream. Remember to add the ingredients of love or joy or happiness with all your might to your dream. Don't hold back and allow yourself to actually receive what you dreamed of. Believe it is already yours and then let go and trust.

You can have a vision board on your fridge, at work, at home, anywhere that is visible. I will take you through the easy steps to create your own vision board and keep your dreams real a little later on.

Visualisation

A visualisation is much like a vision board, except you can change it each time you participate. Rather than getting excited about what you want, it's a way of settling down the body and mind. This is really fun to do at home, in a group, with the kids or on your own. Again, you can make it what you want. Usually, the visualisation is a way to reconnect with yourself and Mother Nature. It uses breathing to quiet the mind and is used to calm an erratic mind. The best way to do this is to sit in a quiet and peaceful place. You will need to make sure you are warm enough and comfortable. To take part in a visualisation, you need to close your eyes. You can use deep and full, slow breaths filling your stomach with air first then allowing the air to spread up to fill the lungs. Keep your breathing controlled and as you breathe out relax each part of your body. After a few minutes of this, you will start to notice how much more relaxed you have become. When you have been in a really busy environment, you will find that it takes you a little longer to properly relax. That's fine. Allow yourself between 10 and 20 minutes at first. After a few minutes of breathing in and out gently, you can start to focus your attention on what you would like to see. As this is a relaxing and reconnecting visualisation, you can picture yourself in a beautiful, lush, green field or by the seaside, or sitting in a beautiful garden surrounded by the most amazing array of heady scents rising up from the beautiful flowers, or on the top of a tall mountain with views all around you. You can imagine yourself to be anywhere in the world that you would find peace. Take yourself through this for a few minutes, just noting what you would see around you. Observe all the wonderful things you can bring into view and how relaxed and at peace you now are. Some people prefer to be led through a visualisation; others find that their own imagination carries them through. You can join a mindfulness group if you like to have someone else guide you through this and other breathing exercises; or you could follow instructions on a CD or on the computer. Although you can visualise before you go to bed, it might be easier sitting up, otherwise the temptation to fall asleep before you have finished could prove too strong. Mindfulness is a fantastic way to help alleviate stress, and will be described in more details later on in the book.

Intention – The Power Of Intention

When you set an intention, you are in effect making a statement to the universe of what your heart desires. When that desire is aligned with spirit, it will be already on its way to you in some form or another. The power of intention is magnified when more than one person shares the same intention at the same time. There have been intention experiments carried out by scientists with a small group of people involved, working together with the same intention, and the process seemed to be quite effective. When you set an intention to do well in the world and a group of people is participating all at the same time, the power is squared by the number of people in that group. So for 1 person, the power is 1. For 2 people the power is 4; 3 people have the power of 9, and so on. So the more people, the more powerful the group. This gives rise to so many possibilities. What if it was your intention to send love to a distant relative? How about sending love to a sick child? What about peace being sent to a troubled area? Wow, that would be powerful. When people work together with a shared interest in helping others and act from a place of love, anything is possible.

To get some understanding of what your essence and the ego are, you need to accept to a certain extent that we are all in fact spiritual beings living in human bodies. To make it easier for you to imagine, visualise there's a little angel on one shoulder and a little devil on the other, like in the cartoons you watched as a child. And in those cartoons, the angel is your spirit, or if you prefer, your essence. The devil is the ego. The ego is like a demanding spoilt brat, seeking constant attention. Its role is to sabotage each and every area of your life. It is the nagging voice that tells you, "You can't do that! Who do you think you are?" It is about as far away from love as one can get. Each time you give the ego attention, or reply to the chatter it creates in your mind, it becomes stronger. Some people have very visible egos and others not so much. People who are most at peace with themselves quite often also have small egos and have mastered ways to keep the chatter at bay. Now the amazing thing is that when you give the ego no attention, it dies down. Be aware, however, because this ego isn't going quietly. The ego will come back when you think you have it under control. Later I will show you ways in which you can quiet the mind and therefore think more clearly.

When you are born, you are pure, unaffected, and eager to learn, happy to be, hungry for life, knowledge and love. Over time, you adopt the view and beliefs of others around you, your family, schools, the environment, religion, and authorities. You take on other people's opinions of you, which may be completely out of line with your own views. The scary point here is that no one is going to let you into this secret and sadly it is something that you have to discover for yourself.

You start to believe what others say about you, taking on their prejudices and living within their limits, making your world smaller. By the time you reach adulthood, there are a lot of layers covering your pureness. If unchecked, there remains a lot of unpicking to do for you to get back to the truth of who you are. In some cases, when the body and mind become unwell, and in cases where people simply feel unable to cope with the reality of their life and have been completely disconnected, the work needed to help these troubled individuals is carried out by the medical profession, therapies or heavy medication. This is what happens when an unbalance in our body and mind occurs.

Now it does seem that this isn't always the case for everyone; there are the odd exceptions. You may be thinking "I lead a charmed life, I certainly have not been affected in this way," then I applaud you; that's great. However, chances are you formed your opinions of yourself a long time ago, probably between the ages of birth and 6 years old. These beliefs or opinions are holding you back. So break the chains and reach your Bliss. There is some work to do. Did you ever hear an adult say "You stupid boy!" or "You are an idiot!" or "Who do you think you are, the queen of Sheba?"

The words you use and the words of others are very powerful; they do untold and lasting damage. This is because you adopt the opinions of others as your own and therefore become restricted by them. The thoughts you think are also powerful; you are powerful. More powerful than you could imagine and yet willingly you have given that power away to live the life that others think you should. The life that others approve of. Learn to be yourself; no one will thank you for behaving like someone else. Be brave enough to stand up and be counted for leading a life of being true to you.

You see, you have done such a great job of programming your own brain into believing that you CAN'T do certain things or have certain things, that it's time to turn that logic on its head. So take the brave step from "I can't" to "I can." You allow your thoughts and other people's words to control you and when those people are amongst those you love and look up to, challenging them is next to impossible, so you have to be taught how.

"If you think you can you are probably right; if you think you can't you are probably right!" Never has a truer word be said.

By learning to change your thoughts, you ultimately change your life. The words you use affect you in subtle ways. Change these in a positive way and your life will be transformed. I think the reason why more people don't adopt this very simple habit has to do with the fact that many are reluctant to change. Most people seem quite happy to accept their lot and therefore don't see the wondrous adventures that could be laid out before them if they only looked up to notice.

There are people who have been in debt, homeless and yet managed to turn their lives around. Do you suppose this was by continuing to put themselves down? No. It was with an innate courage, perseverance and deep-seated desire to improve their lives. Happiness is a choice; what you choose happens. You can decide to be happy and you become so. This is because it's how we have been wired. You all have choices. When you smile, your endorphins, or happy molecules, are released into the brain to make you feel happy – amazing! So along with your positive thinking, smile even when you don't feel like it, and if you do this enough times, you can turn your life around. If others can do it, so can you.

New Daily Takeaway Rituals – This is a powerful practice

This powerful visualisation is a way to reconnect to you, to nature, mother earth and all of mankind.

Sit in a comfortable, quiet and safe place where you are not likely to be disturbed.

Close your eyes and imagine yourself walking in an open and beautiful field. You walk for a while in this field until you reach a tree.

It's a big, majestic, ancient oak, hundreds of years old. This tree has lived a thousand lives and has many secrets to share with you.

The oak is strong and powerful, you feel safe, and so you sit down next to the tree and lean against its vast trunk. The leaves shade your face from the sun and let the heat of the day in.

You feel safe sitting in a lush green field under the tree, surrounded by gorgeous wild flowers, with the sun shining down heating up the earth and you.

You are comfortable, peaceful and relaxed. You breathe in the delicate scent of the breeze. With each breath you breathe in, you take in life-giving oxygen, provided for you with love from the tree.

With each breath out, you imagine releasing everything that no longer serves you. Any negative feelings from your day or week or month, just let them go.

Take a few more breaths like this and as you do so feel the strength of the tree and the enormity of mother earth holding you safely as the earth spins around in orbit.

Imagine that all of humanity is breathing in with you, every baby, child, woman and man. Feel this amazing connection.

Take a few more breaths, now visualize all the animals tame and wild, including the insects and the sea creatures all breathing in and out with you too. Feel that power.

Get Blissed

When you feel completely relaxed and totally connected, take a few more controlled and relaxing breaths, then you can just be. Relax.

Chapter 6
Wellness - Body, Mind & Soul

Make the connection between your body, mind and soul. Flex your body, mind and soul power to see how they are all linked. Your body is connected to your mind and also to your soul. Things don't usually just start to go wrong with your body if your mind is completely healthy and you are eating well and taking care of yourself. Live a life of wellness and kindness. Look after yourself, nourish your soul, do what you love, live your true life's purpose and find your bliss. If you are not clear about what it is that you enjoy or love doing, then pause for a moment and think about what makes your heart sing. What makes you want to jump out of bed in the morning? What is it that makes you feel alive?

Take the time to write down all the things you love to do and all the things you're good at. This list will reveal to you what line of work you need to look at for yourself. Also it will guide you towards how you might want to spend your spare time. When you focus on the things that you enjoy and the things that you are good at, it doesn't feel like work at all. It is more like life with ease. When you start to follow this path, you begin to discover a life of empowerment and joy, and realise that life was not meant to be difficult. Life is an adventure, as well as a series of lessons designed to help you develop and grow.

There is no point in spending your whole life doing something that feels empty to your heart, just because it pays well. Stop doing a job that your parents encouraged you to do for financial security and good prospects. Don't wait until the end of your life to realise that it's been spent doing things that other people expected of you instead of walking your own path. Each of you has a journey to take. The journey of your life. Don't focus all your energy at work climbing the corporate ladder only to find that, when you reach the top, you are on the wrong ladder.

Be true to who you are.

When you spend your time doing the things that you truly enjoy, it fills you up. You start to learn how to live an honest life, a life of authenticity and happiness. Living a life of true abundance is so much more than being financially secure. This is your life, remember, no dress rehearsals here. You can change your life by changing your thoughts, and being prepared to take any action necessary to help you get there. Be brave and have faith in your convictions. Learn to follow your intuition; it is after all your internal satellite navigation system. You just forgot how to use it. Small steps lead to mountains being climbed. Have faith in your convictions, believe in yourself, be true to your heart and live the life you only ever dreamed of.

Eat Well. What type of food?

The food you eat and the drink you enjoy fuel your body. You wouldn't put orange juice in your car and expect it to run efficiently, so why would you not nourish your body with what it needs? There is an undeniable connection with poor diet and poor health. When you choose to fill your body with foods that have little or no goodness in them, foods that have no vitamins or minerals, your body continues to work at the same speed. Your body is an incredible machine that functions at maximum capacity 24/7. When you decide not to give your body exactly what it needs, it will start to take the precious minerals, fluid and vitamins from your muscles and bones. When this happens your resources become depleted and in time your bones and muscles become damaged due to neglect.

For the most part these are very small unnoticeable changes that occur gradually over time, and it is only when the precious resources have all been used up that your body cannot function at this level any more. The rise over the last 30 or 40 years of fast foods from huge food-producing corporations has been repeatedly sold to us as a convenient way of living. We have become seduced by the ready meals culture with the promise that they will feed us quickly and conveniently, thus giving us more time to work and enjoy our lives.

The truth is that these enormous powerhouses that provide all of these ready meals don't really care at all about our health. They only care about their bottom line, profit. Over time, you have accepted the fast food option as a way of life. You have completely bought into it and today, generations on, you don't actually know another way. Sadly, the majority of people don't grow their own fruit and vegetables any more. You more often than not don't prepare fresh meals each day, and rely more and more on a quick snack, a ready meal or fast takeaway food.

I am talking about educated people who need quick and easy meals, so that they can fulfil their working obligations and have a chance to enjoy a social life too. These are the people who train at the gym several times each week to keep fit, not realising that, at the same time, their bodies are not able to cope with the lack of minerals and vitamins and proteins and good fat the body needs to work properly. These are the people who pump their bodies full of protein foods and energy drinks whilst pumping iron at the gym, pounding the streets and aiding their exercise regimes. Are you one of these people? Yes, I'm talking to you.

Do you actually know what goes into these protein shakes and energy drinks? Do you know what is in the body-building supplements you fill your body with, believing that you are enhancing what you have to make the best of it? There are many natural super foods that you can enjoy with no harmful side effects that can assist with physical performance, such as goji berries, green tea, mulberries, bee pollen, wholemeal pasta, brown rice, green vegetables, blueberries, chia seed and spirulina to name but a few.

Whilst a takeaway treat is nice once in a blue moon, it does not mean every few days. The knowledge and ability to prepare and cook yourself a nutritious, healthy meal seems to be largely lost due to the pressurised lives we all lead. Just go into a supermarket and notice what's on the shelves. Notice what the marketers have been providing for you. Notice what the other shoppers have in their baskets and trolleys. Now, I'm not saying that we are all ignorant, not by far, but rather that we are continually being bombarded by adverts and enticements in the guise of making our lives easier by buying microwave meals. That doesn't sound too healthy to me. It's all about the flavour, and in order to achieve the flavours that your pallet prefers, more salt, sugar and fat, as well as unsavoury ingredients are added.

There has been some research recently that showed certain foods, such as ice cream, cheesecake and donuts, to be actually addictive. The reason these foods are addictive and you crave them is because they consist of 50% fat and 50% sugar. Now that sounds disgusting, doesn't it, but apparently that flavour combination is irresistible and so your body craves it. However, the bad news is that these food items are incredibly fattening too.

When scientists recently carried out trials using rats, they were given cheesecake and ice cream as their staple diet. This flagged up some concerning results. In fact, when rats were given any other foods they did not put on weight. And yet when the rats were presented with the cheesecake, they got fatter and fatter. I don't know about you, but I find this piece of research quite disturbing.

Your bodies are designed to eat fresh and raw foods straight from the tree, the ground, or from the seas and rivers. The foods that are going to nourish your body and help it to perform at maximum capacity and be healthy are vegetables, fruit, seeds and nuts. Once a piece of fruit is cut from the tree, it starts to lose its nutritional qualities. The longer it takes for that apple or pear to reach you and to enter your mouth, the less goodness it has. When was the last time you asked the question, "How old is my fruit?", "When were my vegetables picked?", "Where did they come from? ", "What chemicals were sprayed on them during growth?";, "Was the ground they grew in contaminated in the last 200 years?" You simply don't ask these questions when you go to do your shopping in the supermarket or wait for the delivery driver to bring you the food you ordered online the day before.

Fish is incredibly healthy, especially when it's not farmed. Meat is full of iron and other important elements, when it's free range. The sad reality is that still a high percentage of the meat consumed in the UK is pumped full of antibiotics and other chemicals, which in turn end up in the food chain and in your bodies when you eat them. Of course these antibiotics are given to the cattle to fight against diseases. However, no one really knows the damage these chemicals have on your body long term. No one knows if they affect your nervous system, brain synapses or your electrical wiring. The fact is that there has been an increase in childhood diseases such as ADHD, aspergers syndrome and autism in recent years, and one cannot help but wonder where all these new conditions and syndromes are coming from and what is causing them. It is worth asking the question; were these diseases so prevalent in the 1940's, 19050's, 1960's, 1970's? I suggest to you that this is a point of interest and certainly worthy of your consideration.

Whilst contemplating the concerns around food, I understand the challenges of feeding more and more people globally and efficiently. It is an equally good argument regarding the production and supply of mass produced foods. What does concern me is that this comes at such a high price. The price is often paid by the innocent and uneducated all over the world. The premise that, in order for the majority to benefit and survive, the minority must suffer is not a view I share.

Each and every one of you has the same right to be here on this planet, to live a full and safe life. To enjoy a happy and peaceful existence. Yes, I hear you say, that's a utopian ideology, and perhaps it is in some respects. However, there is enough to go round. There is enough for everyone. There are mountains of grain and of food waste destroyed each day globally in some parts of the world, and people starving to death in other areas of the world. That makes no sense at all. It's positively barbaric. The reason that apparently there's not enough food to go around has to do with money, power and greed. The wealth and resources of the world are not shared around. They are not fairly distributed because of the cycle of greed that consumes you, or more accurately the governments around the world that systematically strip the poorer countries of their natural resources to feed the richer countries.

There is fluoride added to your water source. Why is that? There are dentists to monitor the health of your teeth and there is fluoride added to most toothpaste. So why the need to add fluoride to your water source too? Fluoride seems to be added to your water to reduce dental caries which remain a public health concern amongst many westernised countries. As many as 90% of children in education, as well as a high percentage of adults are still affected by dental caries that rot the teeth. They are black in appearance and cause pain, requiring filings.

Water fluoridation prevents cavities in both children and adults. It is estimated that there's up to 40% reduction in cavities when water is fluoridised. The published information stresses that when children drink fluoridised water as well as regularly using toothpaste with fluoride in it, this reduces dental caries. On the flip side, some believe that the use of water fluoridation within industrialized countries may be unnecessary and that caries prevention is kept at bay through the use of toothpaste with fluoride used regularly.

What's Invisible In Your food? What's Hidden In Your Drink?

Have you ever stopped to wonder what is really in your food and drink? Do you always thoroughly read the label of each drink that you consume? Were you aware that if there is an ingredient present in your drink that is under a certain percentage, the law allows for that ingredient to not be listed in the full list of ingredients? This opens the flood gate to abuse in my mind. And hence each and every day, we are not fully informed of the way we are pouring all sorts of unnatural liquids down our throats.

What about restaurants, takeaways and other fast food outlets? What sort of food additives are added to the food and drinks served, that give these tasty dishes such flavours or consistency? When you stop to think about how long a drink lasts, you may wonder what is making it last such a long time. What other components go into your food and drink? When you read the labels on the food you buy over the counter, do you understand what all the names and number represent? No, neither do I.

Recently I bought some cordial for my children from a supermarket chain and when I returned home, I decided to research all the ingredients that I didn't recognise the names of on the label. There were two names that I looked up. To my dismay, there were health warnings attached to one of the ingredients with quite awful side effects. Once I managed to actually find an email address for customer service for this store I sent out my email in the hope the said ingredient was a mistake. I attached the piece of research I had found to the email, to make it easier for the recipient to understand my concern.

After a week when I had heard nothing, I decided to email the store again. This time to my delight an email came back after about a week or so, admitting that they were taking my enquiry very seriously. The email went on to say that although this point was outside of their remit, it would be passed onto someone else who would in fact look into the matter, research it and get back to me. Well, of course I was delighted that this large supermarket was taking such a responsible approach to their product line, particularly as this product was aimed at children. Needless to say that, several months on, I am still awaiting a response. So I decided to take the only action someone in my position can, and voted with my feet. I decided to shop elsewhere.

Exercise For The Body, Self-Care. Be Kind and Gentle To Yourself

Your body is your vehicle for life. It needs to last for many years. Not only that, but you will of course expect it to perform at its peak throughout your lifetime. . So then, why is it that actually taking care of this vehicle, your body, seems so difficult for some? It's the most curious of things really. You neglect your body, don't rest it properly, don't feed it properly, don't exercise it properly and on occasion deliberately abuse it!

In order for your body to last and continue to do the amazing job that it does 24/7, you need to be kind to it, nourish it and generally treat it with respect. It is after all your body, so why wouldn't you? Well, I do understand that in reality, it is not always that straightforward. You may feel anger, resentment, sadness or any number of other emotions towards yourself, based on your upbringing, the environment or the experiences you have endured along the way. And that's okay. The fact that you feel this way is only exactly the same as everyone else does. The truth is that nearly all of you will have at some time in your life a negative feeling about yourself and your body. That's perfectly normal.

However, even though it may be normal, it's really not very helpful. In order to live your life to the fullest and for your body to not let you down, you need to look after it. When you treat yourself and your body with a healthy respect, you begin to value the importance of a good night's sleep. Your appreciate the benefits of drinking plenty of water to cleanse your system, you enjoy the sweet, juicy taste of fresh fruit. When you are kind to yourself it feels good to relax and read a good book, to meditate to create space in your life, or to swim in the ocean to unwind. There are so many ways that you can by gentle and kind to yourself. A warm bubbly bath, a massage, a spa day or refreshing walk in the country on a sunny day. You can find joy in splashing in the puddles in the rain, or running your toes through the sand on the beach.

Self-care doesn't need to be costly or time consuming. It's all about filling yourself up first. When you ensure that you are in a good place first, then you are better able to take care of everyone else, and everyone around you benefits. Your loved ones are better loved when you are whole. Make the time for you, to just indulge in something that you enjoy on a daily basis. It could be simply lying in bed when you awaken and meditating for 10 minutes. You might enjoy getting up half an hour before the rest of your household stirs and take yourself off into your favourite chair with a book and a fresh cup of tea.

It is often the simple pleasures that you don't seem to have the time to just enjoy in the midst of your busy day, week, month or year. Once you adopt a daily practice like this and sustain it for 60 days, it becomes a habit. A ritual of self-care. You will benefit from being more relaxed during your day. Your memory and temperament will improve. You will have more patience. This is because you will no longer feel resentful that you had no time for yourself. You can check in with yourself halfway through the day to see how you are feeling. Just stop and take a few deep breaths and ask yourself how you are feeling. How tense are you? If you are feeling a little anxious, take a few more deep breaths and as you breathe out, relax each part of your body and see how you feel. You can easily do this simple exercise at your desk, in the canteen or in the rest room.

For those of you who have a full hour lunch break and are able to get out of your work environment during the day, take a brief walk to refresh yourself. It is always a good idea to break up your day, if only for fifteen or twenty minutes. This break recharges your batteries and makes your afternoon much more productive. It also gives your body a quick stretch and exercise. You are not designed to sit at a desk all day long and yet most of us still do.

Exercise and Healing For The Mind

Learn to train your mind. The challenges that present themselves to you only help you to develop and grow when they are received wisely. Challenges arise to teach you to solve your problems. The mind is an amazing entity. It is powerful and yet needs to be harnessed. When you fill your mind with knowledge and wisdom that is good and words that are positive, encouraging and kind, your mind will expand, develop and grow in a constructive and creative way. On the flip side, a mind that is filled with judgement, regret, worry and criticism will dry up and become useless.

The voices in your head that keep on playing the same conversations each day will ruin your life if they are left unchecked. You must keep an eye on your mind, treat it like any other muscle, like an errant child, and be disciplined with it. This is the only way to maintain mastery over it. One who seeks knowledge learns something new each day. However, one who is lazy may lose their knowledge. Be mindful of the fact that if you leave the mind to run its own course, without giving it regular instruction, it will become your demise.

So the good news is that there are plenty of healthy exercises to befit the mind and help it stay on course. Just by keeping the mind active with puzzles, quizzes, positive thoughts and stimulating conversation, you will maintain a mind that serves you well. As long as you are in charge of it and not the other way around, it will do its job quite nicely. It is very easy to allow the mind to wander, thinking that you are simply daydreaming, and that is fine for a while. However, when you find yourself in the middle of a full-blown argument in your head, that's a warning sign for you to realise that is not helpful. In truth, this is probably the same debate that has occurred many a time and led to nowhere. The arguments, discussions and voices in your head are the ego taking charge. The mind, or ego, as it's also referred to, wants to be in charge and will sabotage your life if you allow it to. The good news is that once you recognise what is going on here, you can stop it. Simply by becoming aware of what is going on in your head, once you see the ego for what it is, the voices subside, for a while at least. You need to stay on top of it.

Once you master catching the ego at work, by just being aware of when it creeps in and starts to take over, that's the time to stand back as if you are now watching a movie and you are simply the observer. If that doesn't make sense to you, you are not alone. It didn't make sense to me either at first. The only way I can help you to be able to see these things for yourself is when you experience them. Stop reading for a moment and wait. In a few seconds, perhaps even straight away, you will become aware of a conversation starting up in your head. At first it will feel like your voice in your head because you have become so used to it. Listen to what it is saying. Without engaging in a conversation with this voice, simply observe it. Imagine you are listening to the radio and the voice is there. You're not having a conversation, just listening, without prejudice or judgement. That is the voice of the ego and all it wants is your attention. When you are able to allow it to be and not enter into dialogue with it, you will have begun to extricate yourself from it. Beware, however, because it will keep coming back. It will try to engage you in a silly conversation and, before you know it, you're hooked again.

Mastering the mind is a lifelong process. It does, however, get easier with time. The ego you can imagine as a little devil on your shoulder, trying to get you into mischief, leading you astray. To be truly free of it, you need to maintain and listen to your inner voice of calm, or the little angel on the other shoulder,

Get Blissed

your intuition, who never leads you astray. There are many ways you can try to keep the ego at bay. The easiest way is simply by being aware and alert at all times, in the same way as you would when you are expecting a friend to arrive at the door. Your senses are on high alert and you are ready for the bell to ring. So in the same way you can learn to catch it as soon as it starts. As soon as that little voice pops into your head, quietly acknowledge and observe it, without entering into any dialogue and watch it as it fades away. Imagine it is like a cloud in the sky passing in front of your eyes, and now it's gone.

You can replace the negative or disruptive voice in your head with a positive statement or thought. This is a case of good overcoming evil, so to speak. Or you can simply laugh at the ego and imagine it and the conversation it is starting, to be the butt of a joke, or for it to be absolutely ridiculous. So for example, if you are at a party and you are concerned that you may trip up in your high-heel shoes, the ego may come in saying "You're going to trip up and look stupid," so in your defence you may retort back in your head with "Oh yes, I will look completely stupid when I fall over and land on the lap of that young man over there and at the same time knock over the vase which will spill the water all over the floor, creating an enormous river that sweeps everyone out of the room into the street and we'll all end up in the swimming pool that's just been created in the street with boats all around filled with flowers, canapes and champagne."

So you see, by keeping the mind in a good state, it will serve you well. It is powerful and requires taming in order to do this. Your body and mind are amazing and when you begin to understand their capabilities, anything is possible. All you have to do is believe. Imagine it, feel it, believe it and let go and trust.

Intuition

Your intuition is your internal satellite navigation system. The role of your intuition is to help guide you through life. To gently steer you along the path of life. You have a choice as to whether you wish to listen to the ever-so-quiet voice or to go ahead and do your own thing. Of course most of you do your own thing, and it is only when parts of your life seem to take a turn for the worse or start to go wrong that you sit up and take notice. Your intuition will never lead you into danger. You can trust your intuition to lead you on a safe path. What you need to do is listen. This is not as easy as it sounds. And the reason for that is there's a lot of noise going on around you. The noise of your friends and family, the noise of your colleagues at work, the noise of the traffic, the noise of your pets, but most of all it's the constant noise and chatter that goes on in your own head. This is the noise that you need to quiet down. This is the noise that prevents you from hearing your intuition. And the only way to quiet that noise is to stop engaging with it. When you cease to get pulled into the continuous dialogue, you hear nothing. At first it may be for just a second or two. This is enough for you to pay attention and notice it. The awareness of that space is astounding; it gives you such peace, just for a moment. Then it's gone, until the next time.

Once you notice this wonderful space and tranquillity you sense when everything in your head goes quiet, you will want to experience more of it. In time and with practice you can increase your moments of quiet. Meditation will help you with that. Each time you become aware of the lengthy, crazy and recurrent conversations you have in your head, the second you notice them, they stop. This is the point where you have the realisation of what is going on. It's the ego. The ego is the little devil that sits on your shoulder all day long and tells you "Don't do this",

"Don't do that", "Who do you think you are?" and so on. A bit like a deranged parrot. The purpose of the ego is to put you down, criticise you and generally systematically sabotage everything that is good in your life.

Your intuition guides you, helps you and keeps you on the right track. When you become in tune with your intuition, it feels like your guide is by your side. You learn to trust in the direction you need to go. Fear drops away and allows you to have more courage and faith in yourself. You begin to develop an understanding that your life has a path, a journey that needs to be taken, and that journey will be magnificent. It will be exciting and wondrous. It will consist of many lessons and challenges along the way. Challenges that will help you to grow, develop and expand.

Healing For The Body

Your body is incredible. All day and all night it is healing and repairing itself. It does this all the time and without any thanks from you. Your body deserves respect and recognition for the fabulous job it is doing each and every second of the day at keeping you alive. Each time you breathe in air, microorganisms enter the body and some of them try to attack it. All this time you are blissfully unaware of the war zones that rage through your body and defend it. Your body will rally round like a battalion of soldiers to keep your organs safe from harm against any foreign bodies that enter through the nose, mouth, eyes and ears.

Your mouth is full of germs and yet your body is used to them. When you kiss someone, you exchange germs and these germs are then attacked by your own internal defence mechanism in order to protect you. When you sneeze your body is actually rejecting foreign bodies that have entered the body and need to be discarded in order to keep you safe. Your body is amazing. The next time you run for a train, jump up to catch something or turn around suddenly on the spot when someone calls your attention, remember how relentlessly your body is working to ensure you don't have to. Start to thank your body for working so well for you so that you can get on with your life. Your body fully supports you, so you should at least say thank you to it once a day, to show your appreciation. When you begin to appreciate what is important, you receive more of the same.

Your body responds to the care you show it. When you treat your body with respect through regular and enjoyable exercise, you are maintaining it. When you eat a healthy and nutritious diet, you are nurturing your body. When you drink plenty of water, you are cleansing your body. When you sleep and rest well, you are caring for your body. When you laugh, have fun and enjoy constructive and positive experiences, you fill your soul up with joy and bliss. When you meditate, practice yoga or pilates, you are giving your body and mind a wonderful relaxing workout. You are nourishing your body in all of these ways.

Complimentary Therapies

Reflexology, Reiki, Chakras

Reflexology is a lovely, gentle, non-intrusive way to relax the body. It works by applying slight pressure to the feet and is carried out by a practitioner. Reflexology can also be performed through the hands and lower legs. Reflexology is used as a way to clear the flow of negative energy around the body. The tops and bottoms of your hands and feet have nerve endings that are linked to all the other parts of your body. Reflexology can be administered to anyone young or old, with a few exceptions. You will be asked to lie down so you are comfortable and often covered with a blanket for warmth and comfort. This is a very relaxing treatment and a wonderful way to feel peaceful and unwind. Always consult a professional prior to receiving any treatment. Treatment is administered by gently working through each part of the body, from the hands, lower legs or feet. It helps restore the body's natural balance in a holistic way. After receiving a treatment, you will need to drink plenty of water to aid the flushing of the toxins from your body.

Reiki is a form of healing that almost always requires no touch at all. This healing method is a two-way process. The therapist is healing by allowing their energy to pass over to the client. The client in turn needs to be in an accepting frame of mind to thoroughly receive the healing given. Some therapists prefer to gently touch their client as they spread the healing energy over the body of the client. As the therapist's hands move gradually over the body, the client may experience heat or cold. This is perfectly normal and part of the healing process. The therapist can detect your energy levels during therapy sessions and offer advice on ways to re boost your energy if need be.

There are seven main chakras in the body. They represent parts of your subtle body that are part of your very existence. They are non-physical channels through which your life force moves. The seven main chakras are aligned vertically through the centre of the body, along the axial channel. From top to bottom, they are:

Crown Chakra, the colour for this is bright purple, this chakra represents inner wisdom and death of the body, it is seen as a state of pure consciousness and often represented by the colour white.

Third Eye Chakra, the colour being violet or indigo. It represents your intuition and the balancing of your lower and high self.

Throat Chakra, a light blue. This chakra signifies communication and growth through expression, independence, feelings of security, fluent thought and spirituality.

Heart Chakra, green in colour. This represents the immune system, complex emotions, unconditional love, circulation, passion and devotion.

Solar Plexus Chakra, yellow like the sun. This is for digestion, personal power, anxiety and matters of expansion.

Sacral Chakra, orange in colour. This stands for relationships, joy, pleasure and creativity, reproduction, enthusiasm and the adrenals.

Root Chakra, represented by the colour red. This signifies your natural instinct, security, survival, sexuality, stability and sensuality.

When you do a chakra meditation, the aim is to align all seven of the chakras for maximum performance of the body. Your chakras open during a meditation. It is important to close your chakras when you have finished meditating to prevent anything negative entering through these channels. By participating in a chakra meditation the purpose is to open all or at least some of the chakras, by observing which chakra area in the body feels warm. This manifests in the part of the body where the chakra is found and begins to pulsate or throb, or may appear to spin. It is then possible to allow for the other chakras to open. This process cannot be forced and will occur naturally. This sensation is freeing and can sometimes lead to an emotional outburst afterwards, such as crying or a feeling of elation. The process is releasing what the body no longer needs. After a meditation, you will feel very thirsty and need to drink plenty of water.

Healing For The Mind

Mindfulness, EFT, Meditation, Being Present

Give yourself a body, mind and soul workout

Mindfulness is a way for you to be aware of how you are feeling. Ensure that you take time each day for you. Check in and see if you are feeling tense or anxious, and take steps to address this. Adopt regular body scans throughout the day to help you maintain calm. Learn how to use breathing exercises to keep yourself feeling supported and balanced. I will lead you through how to do a body scan later on, it's quick and easy.

The workplace is a pressure pot, where at some point in your week you are going to be stretched or pushed to keep your calm. You need to recognise when this is starting to happen and then take the appropriate action to combat any lasting effects. Once you become mindful of this, there are many ways you can support yourself. The reason that this is so important is to prevent you coming home from work each night with a headache. You may make a bee-line for the vodka, beer or wine to just maintain your sanity. You might reach for a cigarette the second you leave the office. These are all signs that your anxiety levels are probably verging on the unhealthy spectrum. But because everyone else around you is feeling exactly the same, it feels normal. That doesn't mean it's right. We will be looking at exercises to help you in your working day to alleviate tension in your body and mind a little later on.

Protect yourself against negative people, energy vampires. Have you ever noticed that those of you who are upbeat and high energy attract those who aren't? That's great if you want to lift those people to the level of your high energy for a short while. However, do be mindful of their need to suck all the energy from you. You can protect yourself with an invisible bubble that you place around yourself like an energy or deflector shield. For fun, make this bubble your favourite colour. This invisible shield will protect you from energy thieves and also negative words.

It is impossible to consider your body, whilst believing that it is separate from the mind. Or in fact when you focus on looking after your mind and think that your body has nothing to do with it, that sounds like madness. Your body and your mind are connected. Each part of your body works more efficiently when you use it properly. When you look after it, and when you are gentle with it and treat it with respect. When you think that we only really use around 5% of our brain, there's so much more potential for learning, problem solving and growing. When you use your brain, you are giving it a workout, flexing the grey muscles. You exercise your brain when you learn, read, do puzzles or problem solve. This is how you keep it in great condition and how you evolve. By nourishing your mind and soul with loving thoughts and deeds, you are being kind to yourself. Make sure that you align yourself with your true purpose by being, saying, thinking and doing those things which give you joy and help you find your bliss.

Your body is like a high-performance car. It consists of the most sophisticated engineering and is made to last and to be pushed. You wouldn't dream of leaving a high-performance car in the garage, would you? No, you want to drive it, get it out on the road, see what it's capable of and push it to the max.

Over time, when you leave your body in the garage, so to speak, eventually it stops working for you. Like a car getting rusty and seizing up, your body will waste, your muscles will reduce and a layer of fat will build up around your body. Your bodily functions will become irregular and sluggish. Treat yourself every day with a high-performance body treat. This life you lead is meant to be fun, an adventure to be lived, enjoyed and experienced.

Be around positive people, those who make you feel good, those you aspire to. Raise your game. These people can help you step up. . These positive people have moved on from the negative, critical talk and judgement doldrums and entered into the "life without worry class". This is a safe place for you to be and grow and develop, and is a perfect environment for you to expand in. A place to feel supported, to learn and grow.

Show kindness to those you meet. Every day look for ways to offer kindness to others. Kindness opens the heart and mind. It enriches your life. Ask yourself "Am I being kind?" Engage your brain before you speak. You have two ears and one mouth for a very good reason. Take heed, speak less and listen more. When you truly listen to another person, they feel appreciated. You are an energy being and what you give out is what gets returned to you multiplied. The universe loves you and wants you to live a full and happy life.

EFT or emotional freedom technique is an ever-growing therapy used mainly in the treatment of habits and fears. It is immensely potent and the results are both formidable and lasting. The beauty of EFT or "tapping" is that it's simple to learn and can be carried out by a practitioner who is present or remote. The techniques can then be adopted by the clients, who can continue to treat themselves. Top athletes use "tapping" to focus themselves before a race. The results of those who use this form of therapy find that they reach the desired place in a very short period of time.

"Tapping" has been shown to enhance the attention span of pupils at school and therefore makes learning for some students easier. It can also help to calm over excited children and therefore assist with their learning and that of those around them. The knock-on effect of course is that this makes life easier for the teachers too. A win:win situation. EFT does not require a prescription or the use of any chemicals. It is safe and easy to follow. The session does not take a long time, the results are long lasting and much faster than other more traditional forms of therapy. The process shifts blockages in the body that have formed over time. Values that you have held and beliefs you have adopted that have kept you living in a restricted place that no longer serves you. This technique helps you to shift these limiting beliefs you have for yourself.

EFT helps with unpleasant memories through a process known as matrix re-imprinting. The memories you have form your belief systems and values. When these experiences are unpleasant in any way to you, they become belief systems that you subconsciously give power to. By adopting these belief systems, you then spend the rest of your life looking for proof that they exist. For many of you, myself included, this is not helpful and limits the way you live your life.

By recognising these limitations for what they are, and changing them so that they are more in line with your current direction in life, you are able to move forward. No longer will your journey feel as though you are walking through treacle, but more like the flow of the waters in a river. You will feel freer and lighter and more confident with who you are. Some of the limiting views you have of yourself may seem inconsequential, and yet they might have prevented you from applying for that particular job or stopped you from viewing that amazing house because you felt those things were above what you were entitled to in some way. So understanding how you are programmed from an early age, and then realising that you can change that programme, is absolutely incredible. So why not try EFT for yourself?

Meditation is a great way to stop for a brief moment in this busy world we live in. Anyone can meditate, and you can meditate for just five minutes if that's all the time you've got. Meditation is when you sit or lie down, close your eyes and focus on your breathing to relax your whole body. You can focus on your breathing alone or visualise being in a beautiful place, the seaside perhaps or the country, surrounded by nature. You can focus on a colour or flower. You can focus on your chakras. We will be looking at chakras in more detail later.

The purpose of meditation is to stop and rest the mind and body. Meditation helps to train and calm the mind, to focus on nothing or as mentioned earlier something simple like a flower. Meditation is used to combat anger or feelings associated with the negative. The practice of meditation builds your core and therefore strengthens you and helps you feel more grounded. In turn you become more in touch with nature. Some people prefer to repeat a mantra whilst meditating. This is a phrase that's repeated over and again in the head, such as "I bring peace to my life" or something that will help keep the mind focused and prevent it from drifting. It's a form of discipline to focus the mind. Meditation calms the mind and therefore has powerful side effects such as reducing the heart rate, blood pressure and anything else related to anxiety-induced illnesses. The beauty of meditation is that anyone can do it; all you need is a comfortable, warm place to sit where you are not disturbed.

Being present is simply a way of fully embracing the present moment, to relish exactly what you are doing at this precise time. Most of you go on auto pilot when you get up, brush your teeth, get dressed, eat your breakfast, drive to work and so on. You can tell whether or not you have been in this very moment as you look back on your day. Did you ever say to yourself "I don't remember getting home from work" or " I don't recall drinking that cup of tea"? These are perfect examples of when you weren't present. You were away with the fairies, on auto pilot and operating at a habitual level.

When you truly focus on what you are doing right now, enjoy it and embrace what you are doing with vigour, you firstly enjoy the task much more and secondly you are present. So the next time you do anything vaguely dull, like the washing up, decide you are going to focus 100% on precisely what you are doing. Feel the warm soapy water on your hands, the bubbles moving through your fingers, the hard and yet smooth touch of your plates, the soft cloth in the water that floats and turns as you use it to clean off the dirt from your dishes. Even the mundane can be turned into something much more enjoyable. This is what being present does for you. It enhances your experiences of life, even the seemingly dull ones.

Body, Mind and Soul Workout

This is the whole self-concept. You see, it's impossible to consider ailments in the body not relating to the mind when we are totally connected. Likewise, how can we have pain in our souls and agony in our hearts or minds and expect our bodies to not object? For too long we have gone to the doctor, with this pain or that ache and been given a pill. We expect a pill for every ill. And yet, does the doctor ever tell you to go for a long walk in the country, ask if you are sleeping okay, or find out what you eat on a day-to-day basis? Are you ever asked if you are feeling under pressure or upset in any way? Usually not. The physical symptoms are addressed in total isolation from the rest of your being. Unless you treat the whole person, you will never reach a lasting solution.

For headaches you can take feverfew, a commonly grown flower, you can drink plenty of water, and you can run regular mindfulness body scans to relax your body. By identifying where the tension is, you can stand up from your desk and take a wander and in doing so relax your shoulders and give your eyes a break. Each time you stand up your cholesterol goes down, but it's doubtful your boss will tell you that. Most of the illnesses around can be avoided, by taking great care of yourself. By nourishing your mind, body and soul, you are giving it what it needs. Fresh fruit and vegetables, a good night's sleep, regular and fun exercise, as well as staying positive and of course having lots of laughs and good times with friends and loved ones.

When you take care of yourself for even ten minutes each and every day, when you first wake up, you are giving yourself a boost, elevating yourself to a higher level and building up your own resilience levels. This puts you in better health and more able to help those around you in the best way. The people around you will pick up on the vibes or energy you are emitting and respect you as much as you respect yourself. When you neglect yourself by rushing around all the time taking care of everyone else first, you are putting yourself down, adding pressure to your body and sending messages that you are not worth it to your mind. When you start to neglect yourself, others pick up on this and subconsciously follow suit.

So think very carefully, especially the mothers out there, who instinctively put their own families first. Do you want to be respected for practicing a little self-care to prepare you for the day ahead and put on your own oxygen mask first? I for one strongly suggest that you do. Or will you continue to neglect yourself, thinking you are being selfish if you don't put yourself last, and carry on feeling unappreciated, exhausted and unimportant? The choice, as in most matters, is entirely yours. Remember that this could make the difference between feeling great and just getting by. Charity starts at home. This is exactly what those words mean.

When you are in a good place, you are better able to help others without draining your own energy levels and precious resources. Learn to check on how you are feeling throughout the day. Do you feel anxious, stressed, worn out? If so, learn to listen to your body; it gives you the signs. You are all too busy rushing around ignoring the messages your body is giving you. When your body shouts out "Stop!", it is letting you know that you need to rest. All it takes is a quick body scan, (and I will walk you through this later on). You may need a walk in the fresh air, a cup of tea in a quiet place, to close your eyes and just breathe gently to calm yourself down, or do an amazing visualisation. (I will talk you through this technique a little later on too.) By starting to listen carefully to what your body tells you, you will hear the quiet voice that is asking you to stop for a moment, to have a drink, to go for a walk.

Make your body and mind sing by doing stuff you love. What makes you feel alive? What did you love doing when you were a teenager? You may like to go dancing, play tennis, take up running again, and start competing at cycling, horse riding, golf or jumping on a trampoline. When you treat your body to something fun, it feeds your soul.

When you nourish your body with fresh foods and juices and all the delicious ingredients to cleanse, detox and feed each and every organ in your body, your body in turn will thank you.

Your body is amazing. It works tirelessly and constantly without any thanks from you most of the time. Your body continues to do an incredible job, often without all the minerals and vitamins that it needs. When you lovingly nourish your body, every part of it works better. When your body works well, you in turn feel great and your health improves. Nourish your mind with beautiful thoughts and affirmations and make yourself feel great. Say kind words to others and yourself; this will help to make your mind and body align. When you fill your soul with bliss by doing the things that make your heart sing, you are addressing each part of you.

New Daily Rituals - Vision Boards

Having a vision board is a really good way to fast track your way to achieving your dreams!

You can have a vision board on your fridge, at work, at home, or anywhere that is visible. You need to put it in a place where you can look at it each day. This will be a daily reminder to you of what you want in your life. I will take you through the easy steps to create your own vision board and keep your dreams real.

Here's how you make one:

Cut out an old box and use the cardboard on one of the large sides.

Cover one side of your box with all the pictures of everything you ever wanted -- your dream house, car, plenty of money, amazing cuisine, holidays to tropical and exotic places, a pet, some new clothes, your ideal partner or whatever.

There are no rules here.

This is all about your dreams, your desires, so dream as big as you like.

Once you have covered your vision board with all the pictures of everything you can think of that you want to bring into your life, place it in a prominent position.

Look at your vision board each and every day.

Do one for the whole family. Get everyone involved and have a section for their dreams.

See how they all fit together.

It's a great way to have fun with your kids.

This practice also helps you drill down on what's really important to you in your life.

It may be that for you enjoying great health would really change your life.

How about your first home?

Perhaps it's having a child of your own, or being able to regularly give money to charity.

Whatever your heart is capable of desiring is out there for you.

All the possibilities that could ever be are already waiting to be claimed.

There's plenty for everyone.

Chapter 7
Educate Yourself

Question Everything

Why do you accept what you are told? Why do you believe what those in authority tell you? Why do you not question the information you are given when it doesn't resonate with you? Do you trust what the teachers say? Probably. What about the mechanic at the garage who tells you what is wrong with your car? Do you trust him? Would half the work he quoted suffice? What about what the politicians tell you? Do you trust them? There are times, of course, when they are just power hungry and want to keep you in the dark. Can you tell the difference? Do you question their word or accept it blindly just because they are in positions of power? How about what your doctors tell you, when there may be another way? Why not check out "What doctors don't tell you, WDDTY." This is a very insightful website. So, all I am saying here is simply to get educated, be a bit more savvy about what's really going on around you, especially when it affects you. This is the same for your body and certainly your mind.

Bet you love ice cream, cheesecake or croissants, don't you? That's fine; however, do you know why you keep eating foods like these and why you looked forward to having more of them? It's because of the combination of fat to sugar in these dishes. It's 50/50. There are documentaries and books that warn us of unhealthy foods and yet we choose to remain ignorant. We really do make that choice all by ourselves. I don't mean to make you feel uncomfortable here. It is my deep desire to encourage you to use your brain, to flex those muscles in your head and make the best choices you can to support all areas of your life.

It is a fact that when a patient is told by a doctor that he or she is terminally ill and that there's nothing more to be done to help them, the patient will often go home to die. This is a very shocking fact. I have seen it for myself in those I have cared for, and it breaks my heart. And yet, once we discover our inner power, we can turn around and challenge this advice, question it and find alternative solutions. Now I apologise for simplifying this and making out that there is always a silver lining, but, hey, there is, once you take that stand to be totally responsible for your life and to get educated about what is good for you and what is not. Once you throw out of the window what others say to make you feel safe, once you learn to completely rely on your inner wisdom and strength, I promise you will want to know as much as you can to ensure that this life, your life, the most incredible story of you, is the best, most amazing, joyful, purposeful and blissful life it can be.

Challenge and Change

Make it your business to not accept everything you read, hear or see. Take charge of your life and your destiny and make a stand, by questioning, challenging and changing anything you hear that you are not fully comfortable with. Let your intuition be your inner guide. This is how you grow. This is how you find solutions to solve your problems. When you don't challenge and question, you allow those in authority to have far too much power over you. When you are a child, you accept what grown-ups tell you, and to a certain extent that's the right way to be. All children should be able to trust in what the adults around them tell them. Sadly, as we all know, this is not always the case and certainly not always true.

Get Blissed

So then when you reach your adult life, fully qualified to enter the big wide world, most of you choose to continue believing and accepting what you are told. You don't stop to question things that don't make sense to you anymore. Everyone knows that the newspapers and the tabloids put their own spin on stories, depending on whether they are left wing, right wing or somewhere in the middle. It is taken as red that the stories you read about A-listers and such like are mostly to be taken with a pinch of salt. So why don't you question everything else that is printed?

Most of you choose not to challenge those in authority, or even your own friends, for fear of appearing an outsider or someone who wants to shake up the status quo. That's a normal emotion and an understandable feeling for you to have. No one wants to be left out in the cold. But at the same time, when something just doesn't feel right, that's definitely the right time to challenge it. Those in positions of authority know that they won't be challenged by the majority and therefore their behaviour for the greater part goes unquestioned. Of course, most people in positions of authority act in a responsible way. Sadly, however, in certain cases the power wielded by those in authority is not always used for good. If left unchecked it can result in damage caused, which in turn has a knock-on effect on others.

Absolute power corrupts absolutely.

Therefore it is your duty to challenge those around you, especially those in positions of authority. It is a wise man who seeks the council of women. In native America, it was the women and not the men who could vote for the chief of the tribe. Their council was made up of grandmothers, wise women, who put the whole community at the centre. The reason for this was that the strong alpha males understood the dangers of the ego, particularly in the men and understood the wisdom and nurturing characteristics of the women. The women made decisions not based on greed, but instead for the benefit of all. The Declaration of Independence states the document was based on Nature (Mother Earth) and The God of Nature (Father Sky). However, the changes made when the Americans set out to follow the Declaration of Independence was to omit the Nature and hence remove the influence of Mother Earth and therefore the place of women as authorities and guides.

Even with your own friends, it is easy to get led astray by those with a more persuasive voice. This is how gangs are run. There is a clear leader, and then the followers who for the most part follow blindly. It is the birthright of each and every one of you to follow the path that feels right for you. To follow your dreams and desires without others trying to put you down or hold you back. It is breaking the barriers that stand in your way that I am trying to get you to recognise, so that you in turn can be clear of the road you want to take, and take it feeling good about yourself.

You are controlled by power and yet you say you want to be free. Freedom is knowledge and taking charge of yourself. You trust what your parents say, you trust what the teachers tell you, you trust what your dentist, doctor, accountant, policeman and politicians say to you. When you are told by your doctor that you have depression and he writes you a prescription, do you question the doctor or trust him? Well, you trust him or her of course. But why? Do you ask the chemist what's in the medication prescribed? Have you any idea what the side effects of all the pharmaceutical drugs are that you are taking? If not, why not? This is your body you are ingesting these chemicals into. Start to question, challenge and change where you need to. Get educated; there's a wealth of information at the touch of a button, so for our generation and the next and the last, knowledge is easy to come by, thankfully. Become more savvy about the world around you. Knowledge is just education. Make sure you become educated in the areas of your life where you are currently not. If you have to take pharmaceutical drugs, then look into the ingredients, the side effects, how extensive the drug trials were before they were brought to market. What are the alternatives? Are there holistic drugs you could have with fewer side effects? Are there any other people who have overcome your ailment or condition that have not used pharmaceutical drugs? Could you be cured by simply changing your diet, drinking more water, getting more exercise, getting 8 hours sleep each night and leading a really healthy life? That's a really good starting point.

You see that when you take medication regularly and you take it because of a serious condition, you get scared of what may happen if you miss a day, or stop taking that medication full stop. You fear the worse and think you will get sick or even die in some cases if you stop taking it. This is a very true fact. The drugs you take end up controlling you. You feel your power slip away through your fingers. You somehow feel that, unless you have this medication, you won't survive. That is a dreadful place to be and so I urge you to question, challenge and change. Do your research. Find out what your options are. Look outside of the pharmaceutical sector. Broaden your horizons. Get educated. Learn how to best take care of yourself.

There have been cases of cancer patients increasing their vitamin C intake up to 100,000 milligrams per day to help their own natural immune system to fight the cancers. There have been people who have gone to Mexico to receive a treatment that wasn't available in the UK or America. The treatments that these people have found for themselves have changed their lives, empowered them to take back control of how they treat their own bodies, and they have recovered.

Now of course I understand that we put so much faith into the medical profession and I am in no way suggesting that you shouldn't put your trust there. The medical profession and the NHS in the UK do an incredible job. Of course they have their place. It isn't the doctors and the nurses, and the consultants and the surgeons that need to be avoided, but rather the enormous powerhouses that are the pharmaceutical industries who make so much money and who are so far removed from "care" that their focus is world domination and making money.

Doctors do not receive much training in nutrition; that's a fact, so they are not the best people to advise in this area. A nutritional therapist will spend a minimum of 3 years studying foods and being out in the field carrying out case studies. They will study in detail the impact those foods have on the body, so for expert nutritional advice, that's where you need to start looking. In fact with any ailment, that's where I would start to look. What does your diet look like? Your sleep patterns, exercise, lifestyle and so on.

You see, when you have a pain in your shoulder, you traditionally visit the doctor. The doctor will look at your shoulder, ask you some questions and either prescribe a pill or refer you for an x-ray at a hospital. However, if you instead went to visit a sports therapist or body and muscle specialist, they would look at your whole body posture. You would be asked a hundred questions around your work and home life, your sleep patterns, your exercise, your daily routines, any past accidents or operations, your diet and so on. At the end of a verbal and physical examination you would have some exercises recommended to you, and perhaps a further visit. It might transpire that the shoes you have been wearing have had a knock-on effect on the way you walk, which in turn has affected how you stand and hold yourself, and that has affected your posture, which has resulted in the way you hold your upper body, which has ended up causing this discomfort in your shoulder.

So, in fact you have become completely out of line and your shoulder is not in alignment with the rest of your body. This is just an example to show you that when the doctor treats the shoulder in this case, it's not the shoulder that actually needs to be fixed. It's the purchase of a supporting pair of shoes that is required. The doctor won't necessarily reach this conclusion as he is not a chiropractor or sports therapist, he is a general practitioner. Therefore, do educate yourself as to where to start looking, when something goes wrong in your body. And remember that it is your body.

Surround Yourself With Greatness

Make a decision to be around positive people. Spend your time with others who understand and appreciate you. They lift you up. Beware of the energy vampires who drain your energy and go on to the next victim. You may find that, as you become more aware, certain people are attracted to you, whilst you repel others. This is normal and part of self-awareness. Is it really helping you being around those who judge, complain and criticise you? Does it aid in your personal growth? It may be difficult to avoid such people if you work with them, or even live with them. Are you living with the enemy? Is the enemy you? Do you need to make changes in your life to be a better person? There are techniques you can adopt to protect against those who bring you down. See the chapter on mindfulness for more guidance here.

Spend your time around those who make you feel good about yourself. Those who accept you for who you are. Spend your time surrounded by people who share the same values as you do. They will raise your energy levels. Birds of a feather, flock together. You know a variety of many amazing people and that is cool. Make sure that their values are aligned with yours. When you make the decision to improve your life and be the best you can be, having positive people around you can help that happen more quickly. You will find over time that the negative complainers in your life lose their appeal to you as they start to bring you down. There may come a time when it seems right to spend less time with these people because they simply don't satisfy, they zap your energy. When this time comes, just allow for them to fall away as your relationship with these people has served its purpose and now it is time to let go.

When you surround yourself with others who operate on a higher level, who are encouraging and motivating and inspiring, you lift yourself up in the process. When you fill yourself up first, you are better able to serve others. When you are in a space of learning and discovering, it allows you to expand and grow. From this point you are better able and more equipped to live at your highest self and be the best you can in each and every area of your life.

Educating Yourself Takes a Lifetime

Educating yourself is your birthright. It is your responsibility. It is completely up to you to get educated, to find out and equip yourself for life. Spend time at the library or on the computer to do research about any given topic you feel out of your depth with. This will educate you and at the same time empower you. When you understand how your body works, or how your dishwasher works, or how your car works, or what's in the foods you eat and what chemicals they have been treated with, or the impact the chemicals in your cosmetics have on your body, or why you shouldn't allow the dentist to put metal fillings in your mouth, or what's really in your prescribed medicines, then you can make smart informed decisions as to whether you wish to accept these things or take action in your life to change some of them.

You may decide that to sign up for an engineering course would give you the knowledge to service and do the MOT for your car in the future. This would make you feel great about your ability to not have to rely on someone else and at the same time save you the money you would have otherwise paid to a garage. You may choose to carry out some research to look for a company that sells only 100% organic cosmetics. This puts you in the driving seat of what goes onto your face and body and what also gets absorbed into your body and system. These products might cost slightly more, but your skin and your body will be healthier as a result, and you will have complete certainty that you know what is going in to your body and skin. You may make the decision that finding an organic dentist is now a priority in your life. But until you become aware that not everything is as it seems, and educate yourself, you can never take the right course of action for you. And the action that you take of course will be different for everyone, because we are all different.

What one person needs to have a healthy body will be different from the next. Those who suffer from migraines will find that certain foods could be avoided to help alleviate the symptoms, such as red wine, chocolate, tomatoes and cheese. Even this is pretty standard advice, and there are also other causes of migraine headaches too that will need to be examined. The amount of water drunk, the amount of sleep enjoyed, the level of stress in one's life and so on. There are many specialists in this field. Once you begin to search on the internet for healthcare specialists or alternative and complimentary remedies, you educate yourself. Approach companies such as Holland and Barratt who are reputable suppliers of herbal remedies, and you will find that there is a whole hidden world of knowledge and expertise out there.

Whatever it is that doesn't feel right, whether it be in your head, heart, soul or body, listen to what it is that you need. Listen to your body, examine how you are living your life and ask yourself the question, is there anything else I can do to make things better for myself? And if the answer is yes, then run with it. Find out. This is your life. This is your body and what you choose to put into it, body, mind and soul has got to be your choice. Take charge and be in control; it's up to you.

Nature Verses Nurture

Are you the way you are because of the way you were brought up? Are you the way you are due to the environment? I suggest to you that environment has a huge influence and unless you are strong and can overcome its pull, you will get swept away into the rivers of sameness. It takes regular discipline and daily self-control to keep you on your path. The path that will lead you to greatness and enable your dreams to come true.

How much influence does nature play in how you develop, think and grow? Are you the product of your genes, or your parents, or the environment you are brought up into? When a child is adopted at birth, they take on the persona of the family that adopted them. When this is a lovely and nurturing family, that child will flourish. Where the environment around them is hostile, this will also affect the child. So actually, what seems to be the case here is that the environment you are in, the nurturing you receive, has more effect on the way you will turn out as adults. The influence that nurture has over you is stronger than nature. You adapt to the world around you and therefore you evolve.

Get Blissed

Evolution is the process through which you survive. In order to survive, you are required to adapt to your environment. It is only when the environment changes at a faster pace than you can keep up with that you fail. This is what has happened throughout history with certain species of animals. When the environment changed more quickly than they could, they died out, became extinct. In the same way, you must equip yourself in order to develop and grow with the knowledge you need to better your life. So educate yourself, give yourself more power and control and accept that you as well as everyone else is amazing and unique. If you want to be in the driver's seat of your life, you need to ensure that you have the answers for yourself.

When a young person is drawn into a group that is not wholesome and into drinking, stealing or drugs, the environment will win every time, unless that teenager has already put in place the desire to question, challenge and change. Where the seed has already been sown as to the possibilities being infinite for that young person, survival is assured for them and escape is imminent from the gang that is pulling them in. However, where the seed has not been sown and the possibilities in life have not been acknowledged or realised, in almost all cases, that same teenager will eventually succumb to the dark side of the gang. This is the reason it is so important that children are educated at home and at school, and shown that each and every one of them has the chance of greatness. Each and every one of them has the opportunity to become and achieve whatever they want. All they need is to believe in themselves and gain as much knowledge to help them get there. The minute you take charge of your life and say, "This is my life, I am responsible for myself and my future in every way," you are setting the intention of what is in your heart, or your desire, and you have taken the first step to realising your dreams.

New Daily Rituals

This is a fantastic meditation to help clear all the negativity out of your system and fill up your energy levels.

First ensure you have a good 20 minutes of peace and quiet where you won't be disturbed.

Either sit comfortably or lie down in a warm, relaxing place.

Make sure your whole body is feeling supported and your muscles feel at rest.

Bring your attention to your breathing.

Take in 3-5 deep breaths.

As you breathe in, allow your stomach to expand first and your chest last, so that you take in as much energising and life-giving air that you can.

Breathe gently and slowly.

As you breathe out imagine that you are releasing all of the tension that has built up over the course of the day. You feel peaceful, safe and secure. You are held in this space by the universe; you are loved.

Once you have completed your deep breathing, to get you into a fully relaxed state, you can allow your breaths to return to normal.

Now with each breath to inhale, imagine that you are breathing in white light. This light is bright and pure. This light has healing properties and is bathing your whole body in peace and love.

As you breathe in, and with each breath, this bright light flows through each part of your body, bathing it in love and peace.

You are feeling light and safe, you are held. You are healing and your energy flows smoothly around your body.

With each out breath, imagine that all negative thought, any pain and the worries and tensions from your day are being washed up into a grey cloud and swept out of your body through the air in your lungs.

This feeling of purifying your whole body is immensely powerful and releasing. You feel light and free with each breath that you take. You feel safe and secure and connected with mother earth and the universe.

Hold yourself in this space for as long as you feel comfortable. You may drift off to sleep. You may go into a deeper and more cleansing meditation.

When you are ready to come around, take a few deep breaths and allow yourself to stretch if you want to and stay for a moment.

See now how you feel. Have yourself a glass of cool refreshing water to help any toxins leave the body. You are now refreshed and cleansed.

Chapter 8
Stop Watching/ Reading Negative Stuff

What Do You Watch, Read, Say and Listen To?

You take it for granted that the TV, the newspapers and books that you read are for your enjoyment and pleasure. They are there to educate, entice, entertain and inform you. What you might not realise is that everything you read, watch, hear, think and say affects the way you think. What you think affects how you act and, ultimately, what you think changes your life. We take it for granted that the thoughts we think have nothing to do with the direction our lives are going. However, the thoughts we think, what we read, listen to and the words we use are all very powerful, and they create our future. When you watch or read the same genre, you begin to think in the same way that the book or film intended.

So, for example, if you love to read murder mystery books and only read those types of books, the way you think will over time become aligned with the way the books are written. You may start to have nightmares or become a little paranoid and feel unsafe at night. If you only ever watch the news and the 24-hour news programmes and never travel abroad to experience first-hand what the world looks like from the point of view of a traveller, you may start to believe only what the news channels present to you. In other words your world becomes very one-sided. Your view of the world is dictated by what is presented to you on the news, in the newspapers and in the books you choose to read.

When you listen to the same radio channel, your views become aligned with those of the reporters and presenters that you listen to. Now there's nothing wrong with sticking with what you enjoy, so long as you remain aware that there are many other points of view. When you meet different people, travel around the world and read many different types of books and educate yourself, that's when you see the world from many angles, and your world becomes a much more interesting place. You become more accepting of other cultures, religions and ways of life, and realise that we are not so different from each other after all. The world is a fascinating place. It's a place of wonder, adventure and many experiences. It's a world of challenges that help us learn, develop, change and grow.

The words you use have power, as they act and affect you on a subconscious level. When you are told time and time again that you are lazy, stupid, naive or whatever, on a subconscious level, these words hurt and if you are told enough times, you start to behave as though you are what you are being told. Therefore, it is vital that the words you use are chosen carefully as they will in turn affect how another person feels. The words you use to speak with yourself out loud or in your head will also have an impact on how you feel about yourself. Once you become mindful of this, you will automatically start to think before you speak. You can use self-talk as a positive and motivational pastime. Such as encouraging yourself, for example "You are strong, you are courageous!" When you repeat this mantra, or others like it, over and over, your subconscious hears these positive words and responds by making you stronger and more courageous. In other words, if you think you can, you are probably right. On the flip side, when you believe you can't, you are probably right. So it's up to you to decide whether you can or cannot.

What I'm trying to get at here is that we have much more power than we realise. We have the power to change our lives into anything we want, so long as what we desire is aligned with our core or spirit. When we truly believe we can do something, all that is required is for us to get out of our own way so that we can reach our goal. It is not failing when you come second in the race. It is only when you give up at the first hurdle and become filled with fear to start over. When you get up and try again until you win, you are a winner. It is perseverance that keeps us going. When you show up and never give up, it is perseverance that keeps you on track. Winners may lose at times but they never give up. Winner mentality means that each time you fall, you get back up. You only have to look around at the thousands of successful people in the world to recognise that the athlete, the climber, the formula one driver or the business man has had to start from somewhere. Lord Sugar came from very humble beginnings and yet he always turned up; he had that winner mentality and he persevered, no matter what.

In life you may fail from time to time, but at least you tried. In life it is deciding what you want and making the decision to have those positive thoughts in your head that are aligned with what you want. It is to surround yourself with positive role models and mentors who can support your dreams. It is reading, listening to and thinking the right information to support the direction you want to go in, and it is keeping your focus and persevering along the road you know to be the right one for you. When you read, watch, listen to and think the thoughts that resonate with you and the life you wish to live, a shift starts to occur. The direction of your life and the road you choose becomes a little clearer. When your focus is on a wonderful life that you know you want, just like the satellite navigation system in your car, you realign with each step you take. When you begin your journey, you know where you want to go but you don't know every road that you will take in order for you to get there. Trust that your internal guidance system will take you there.

In the same way, you need to set your intention of where you are going, stay focused and mindful of your journey, then let go and trust that one step at a time is all that's required of you. Each time you reach a metaphorical road block, T-junction or roundabout, you simply assess which path will take you closer to your end goal. If necessary you realign yourself. Once you push yourself, you begin to realise what you are capable of. When you discover what you can do, that becomes your driver. When you reach the end of a day that went badly for you, remember that every day is another opportunity for you to start afresh. Every day is the first day of the rest of your life. So if yesterday you felt like you failed at something, today you can start over. Your thoughts are powerful; make them count.

You Are Programmed

From a very early age you are programmed to do the right thing, say the right thing, behave in a certain way, do as you are told and so on. At school you are taught that this is right and that is wrong. You are punished when you deviate slightly, and you are kept on the straight and narrow. At work you toe the line to keep on the right side of your boss. In the pub you behave like your friends do in order to fit in. You do what the doctors tell you and take your medicine, follow the way that the policemen instructs you, and you probably abide by what your husband or wife expects of you. You even follow the politicians when they roll out their spin on how you need to be living your life. There are so many expectations on all of us throughout our lives, and there are also so many controls. It is these controls that keep most of us institutionalised.

The good news is that we can all do something about it should we choose. Change your programming and the thoughts in your head and change your life. When you keep your focus every day on what you do want in your life, that's exactly what you will attract into your life. Give what you want all your attention, every day. Thinking about what you desire once is not going to manifest it into your life. You need to continually do it, think it, feel it, believe it. You need to build the momentum to give those positive thoughts power. When you add a positive emotion such as love, joy, passion to your desires, that's when you add the rocket fuel to accelerate your manifesting what you want into your life. "Be careful what you wish for" has never held so much truth.

It doesn't mean we have no control, because when we challenge and question what doesn't serve us in our lives, we can understand and find ways in which we can change it. Most people seem happy with their lot and that's just fine, but if you, like me, are not one of those people and feel that you have a greater purpose in life, then start to take the first small steps to take charge of your life.

Whether this is the first time you have ever challenged your belief system or not, that is fine. Your belief system is set at an early age in the home. Naturally, we adopt the values and beliefs our parents held, as that's all we know. It's only as we grow into adulthood that we begin to see how some or many of these values just don't serve us anymore. At this point, it's a good idea to challenge them and break free from the mould and the barriers that have held us in that space for so long. Once you de-programme yourself, so to speak, and let go of the beliefs you grew up with, you begin to feel free and liberated. This is when you understand that to be yourself and not what others expect of you is the only way to live.

You Believe What Everyone Tells You

When you are told enough times that you are stupid or that you can't or shouldn't do something, or that you're not good enough, those words hurt and eventually if they continue, they have an effect on how you view yourself. Words are powerful and, when they are used against us like this, they cause us damage. The tragedy is that, most of the time, the damage is permanent and forms our belief system. Unless checked this can remain with us for the rest of our life. From first-hand experience, it has made me stronger and more resilient. As I have gone from a place of being on my knees, I want you to know you can get through any negative beliefs you have been carrying and break through those limiting values that have been holding you back. Energy flows into what you put your focus on, so focus on your self-worth rather than someone else's take on it. Don't allow what others think of you to hinder you living the life you want. Remember that what you focus on in your life will come into view, be it consciously or subconsciously.

At times it is difficult to remain strong and stand in your own power, but you have to find ways of protecting yourself against what other people say about you. Let them think what they like; you know who you are. Remember that what other people think of you is none of your concern. Other people like to judge and criticise, but this is your life, so live it as yourself. Now I know as well as you do that words can really hurt and affect the way we feel about ourselves when they are unkind words. This is why practicing mindfulness (as described in another chapter) really works and will strengthen your core. The techniques given at the end of each chapter will help you when you are in a negative situation. Make sure that you practice mindfulness each day, even if it is just for 5 minutes to do a body scan (described later).

You Are Conditioned

Throughout our lives we are to some extent or other conditioned. Over time we almost become institutionalised, like sheep following the herd as we lose sight of our individuality. The good news is that we can change the fact that we are conditioned. In order to change our conditioning, which is similar to programming, we need to fully focus on what we do want that is aligned with our true self. Any time a negative thought creeps into your mind, banish it, watch objectively whilst it passes by like a cloud in the sky, but never give it attention or power. If you do, it will detract from all of your positive thoughts. When negative thoughts enter your head and you engage with them, what you are trying to manifest into your life becomes like a seesaw, two steps forward, one step back.

In other words, you move from positive to negative and so on, and you end up going nowhere, as the two cancel each other out. Remember, your thoughts become your reality. In order for your thought process to become strong you need to keep up a positive momentum. By exercising your mind in the same way as you would any other muscle, it becomes stronger. Over time, and with daily practice, your thoughts will change automatically to ones that support what you want. However, at first it takes discipline to get out of any old habits of doubt or negative thoughts sneaking in. Make a vision board that you keep in a prominent place and look at each day. Regularly adjust and add to it accordingly. When you manifest something from your vision board into your life, make sure you acknowledge that, be grateful, feel delighted. Keep a journal and write down 10 new things each day that you're grateful for and why.

Make sure you remain in the company of those who fill you up, inspire you and motivate you. Avoid people who drag you down, judge you and suck your energy from you. These people will pull you down and hold you back, and force you to become like a conditioned sheep instead of striving to become who you really want to be. Find a mentor to guide you to your next goal. Look for someone who can help you to the next stage of your life in whatever area you feel you need that extra leg up. Keep your focus on the long-term goal and don't get caught up in the details. At the same time, don't worry about the journey, your inner guidance will get you there. All you need to do is to keep on the right track. So every now and again you may need to slightly adjust your course, like a ship on the seas. Be aware not to lose sight of your end goal and keep your focus. Enjoy the ride because that's part of your journey, and no doubt there will be lessons to be learned along the way. Don't lose your nerve when times get tough. Instead, reassure yourself that this is just a road block and you can walk around it or climb over it. Keep your eye on your true prize as well as enjoying the view. Your life journey is an adventure to be enjoyed and savoured.

When making changes in your life and de-conditioning yourself, keep a journal and write down each morning 10 things that you want. Say your daily affirmations out loud to help you manifest them. Just before you go to bed, repeat them to yourself, preferably out loud, or write them down. Then as you sleep your subconscious will work to help bring them to you. If you like to keep notes on your laptop, mac, iPad or other device, they can be stored as a daily reminder that can prompt you at the start of each day. You can then amend your list accordingly.

Is Your Creativity Being Suppressed?

When you're busy rushing around and don't give yourself any head space or "you time", your creative juices dry up and become blocked. We are all under such pressure to just keep up, let alone get ahead. Most of us have little or no spare time and when we do there's usually a gadget attached to us taking our attention. Sometimes it's self-induced and sometimes it's because our boss expects us to be on call 24/7. Either way, we seem to have lost the ability to just be, rather than do all the time. In fact, we feel that if we are not busy doing something, we are wasting our time or being unproductive. This is an illusion and is causing us to feel suppressed. We end up suppressing all our creativity and start to believe that we are not creative. We are all creative in different ways. You may be artistic, a singer, dancer, painter, writer, actor or creative with textiles or bricks, Lego, jewellery or dressmaking.

Give yourself a break; take the time to go for a walk or just sit quietly and have a cup of tea without talking, reading, texting or speaking with someone. Give yourself time to think, time to be and time when you don't feel the need to be attached to a screen or device of some description. We are running on auto pilot most of the time as the pressures of life run rings around us, and so we end up missing out on smelling the roses, appreciating the birds singing, the sound of the waves crashing and the leaves rustling in the breeze. This is damaging our creative side and suppressing it. What are you going to do about taking time for yourself to reconnect with your creativity?

You may find that taking up a new hobby or sport helps bring out your creative side. You might go back to a hobby that you gave up when you started work, got married, had children. You could take a shower, meditate or sing in the rain to help give you time to think. It certainly will help to balance your life. I took up running in my forties, which to my surprise, I really enjoy. You could be more adventurous and take up sky diving, snow-boarding, go-carting, flying or whatever takes your fancy. But choose something that makes you feel alive, that takes you out of yourself and fills you up. I bet you will start to feel more creative and happy at the same time.

Can You Change It All Around?

At first this may seem like a really big deal, but the only way to climb the mountain is by taking one step at a time. To stop the chatter in your mind, to balance your body, to strengthen your core, to allow for space inside of you, are all ways in which you can treat yourself. Why are we all so busy, and insistent on being engaged at all times? We seem not satisfied with sitting in a car, bus, train, plane and relaxing, unwinding, just being. We demand to be stimulated at all times by sounds, images, food, drink, entertainment, and so on. These distractions are not as healthy as you may think. These outside stimuli deflect from you just being and recharging your mind. When you do give yourself permission to stop and get a moment of clarity, it is the most amazing feeling. You feel as if the world has just been paused and you can see it. I mean really see it. You notice that the leaves on the trees seem clearer, more vibrant, distinct, and sharper. You become incredibly creative. There seems to be no effort in forcing out an idea, as it just pops out of your head.

Our bodies are designed to deal with stressful situations. As the stress rises in us, our bodies take the strain. Our bodies can handle even severe stress so long as it isn't prolonged over a long period of time. Our bodies cushion the blow, so to speak, then soften when the stress subsides. What happens in most of our lives, in society at large and in the western world, is that for the most part, our bodies and our minds are not returning back to normal following a stress episode. Therefore, over time the stress hormones build up in our body and make us sick. People who don't have a survival tool box or mechanism in place to use and help the mind and body return to normal tend to get more serious illnesses as they get older. For some, the signs start to show much younger. Those who suffer strokes and heart attacks could be helping themselves and thus reducing their levels of anxiety, by taking mindfulness classes, adopting daily mediations at home, or learning yoga or Pilates. There are many ways to help oneself. Our bodies are connected to our minds, and what we think ultimately creates our life as we are all made up of energy. You can see it in some people when they have lots of energy. It can be measured and scientists can take a picture of your energy with a special camera. When energy gets blocked around the body it ceases to flow freely. These blockages then can cause minor problems that, if left unchecked, turn into bigger problems affecting your health, and in certain cases can bring you to a grinding halt.

Please understand that what I am sharing with you is born out of a deep love that you too can change your life by making a few easy changes, most of which will cost you nothing. I am trying to illustrate to you that by having a metaphorical tool box to carry around with you each day that supports you, it will make a huge difference to your quality of life. We are not meant to spend our time on earth to live alone. We are not meant to feel unheard. We are not meant to feel unhappy. Once you begin to understand who you are, why you are here, what your gifts are and how you can harness them to enrich our lives and others too, everything changes.

If you want change, you need to change.

New Daily Rituals

This is easy and fun to do with children.

Sit or stand. You can do this anywhere.

Rub your hands together as fast as you can until you can feel them becoming really warm. Continue until they feel hot.

Then hold your hands slightly apart so that they are not touching, about 1 to 1.5 inches of separation between them.

Feel that warmth between your hands.

Gently move your hands slightly closer together and then slightly more apart, very, ever so slightly and very slowly so that it feels as though there is something in between your hands pulling them and pushing them.

When you can feel this, you will then know that this is your energy. This amazing energy is what we are all made up of. It is powerful.

This is a simple way to show you how powerful you are and how much energy you have.

When you have an aching knee, arm, shoulder, neck, you can do this exercise of rubbing your hands together, and then straight away place your energised hands onto the area that needs soothing. You will be able to feel this heat, this energy going into that area of your body.

The same method can be applied to children. You can show children how to do this, it's really fun. You can also use this to help comfort and heal your children. And once they can also follow these instructions, it will empower them to do the same for themselves. When they stub a toe, or bash an elbow, you can show them how to relieve the pain and you can help too, to make them feel calm and safe again. What a lovely gift.

Chapter 9
Awareness

Life is a mirror. When you act with kindness, love and respect, that's what you will get back and what you see. When your behaviour is unkind or selfish, that's also what you will find. To live a life of true Bliss, strive to be:

- authentic
- attentive to others
- grateful
- courageous
- compassionate
- charitable
- gracious
- enthusiastic
- kind
- inspirational

When you perform an act of kindness just because you can, your heart lifts. It fills you with joy. Do something today for someone else, without even thinking about it. Say hello to a stranger, buy a bag of fruit for a homeless person. Donate some clothes or toys to a charity or set up a direct debit to support your favourite cause. Living a meaningful life of purpose makes you feel happier and also makes you healthier too. When you give and don't expect anything in return, wonderful things are attracted back to you like a magnet.

Intuition

Your intuition is a gift, a guidance system to help you through life. When you stop to listen, you will notice you often have what's called a "gut feeling" about something or someone. Deep down in your heart, you know whether something is right or wrong, whether it is in line with your true life purpose. You still have a choice, whether in fact you follow your intuition or ignore it. The discussion that plays almost constantly in your head is simply the ego and your soul fighting it out for supremacy. They are having a tug of war most of the time. Ultimately, you need to decide which part of you to follow. It's like the angel on your one shoulder and the little devil on the other. A word to the wise, your soul or essence will never take you into danger. Your ego on the other hand will lead you into mischief and trouble, because that's its nature. Once you realise and accept this, you are in control of which path you take. Don't be scared to step into your own brilliance.

Be aware that the small voice in your head, your intuition, can only be heard when you are still. Even though your intuition is your internal guidance system, for years you may have ignored it, so learning how to really listen again takes time. Have an open mind, allow yourself to relax and unwind. Create space in between those thoughts and then you will hear. The good news is that, like most things, listening to your intuition gets easier with practice.

The more we notice what's going on around us, the more we become present to each moment. When we start to listen, more wisdom comes from our intuition. In the beginning, the messages coming from our inner self may be vague, like a subtle suggestion. In time, they will become more detailed. The messages you receive may not make sense at first. Trust that gradually, the truth for you will unfold. You may find that keeping a journal helps. Write down what comes into your head, even though it may not seem significant at all. Some people see colour or images, symbols or a feeling. Hold onto the pieces and in time, you will join the dots, to form a picture, like magic.

To help you follow your intuition and develop this amazing skill, you need to believe and trust that you are being guided from a point of deep wisdom to help you on your way. If you don't pay attention to the messages coming your way, you could miss out on a fantastic opportunity. When the left brain speaks, you tend to get logic, words. The right side brain is more holistic, colours, feelings, etc.

Sometimes what comes into focus is via another person, an earth angel. They may come along from nowhere and say something that completely makes sense. Remember to thank them for this little gift. A book may fall off the shelf in the library that turns out to be relevant to you, or someone may suggest a book to you. Have you ever gone to send a text to your friend only to find that they are sending you a text at the same time? That's intuition. Have you ever gone to make a phone call only to find that the person at the other end answers immediately, knowing it would be you? This is intuition. You hear of stories where a twin has fallen sick and even though their twin may be far away, they can feel the pain and they rush to get in touch. Did you ever feel someone you care for in your heart and know they are also thinking about you? This is intuition, and is a skill that can be developed and finely tuned.

You can summon your intuition if you need clarity with a certain area of your life. When you ask the question to the universe, "What is it I need to learn today?" you can seek guidance for a problem that requires solving by asking for it. Be specific when you ask the question and see what occurs during the day.

Sometimes you will get a clue from your intuition that makes no sense, so ask another question, "What does this mean?", to get some clarity. You need to listen carefully and piece together the parts of the puzzle. It may take time to join the dots.

You may be very open to listening and even have the gift of being psychic. You might find that angel cards help you uncover the secrets of your inner wisdom. The purpose of using cards is to get you out of your left brain, away from the ego and into the quiet space of listening.

Awareness of Yourself and Others

Being aware is making the most of each and every second. Living life in the moment and valuing the present time, right now, is all we ever truly have. Notice how it feels when you completely give yourself to this moment. Next time you are doing the washing up or cleaning the car, make a point of totally focusing on what you are doing. Don't allow any thoughts to enter your mind. See how it feels. The space in between the thoughts is what allows your creativity to flow. By being fully aware of what is going on around you helps you appreciate the beauty around you. You notice the flowers, birds flying in the sky and the sunset much more when you are fully aware.

Next time you go for a walk, lift your head up and really see what it looks like out there. You may be surprised at what life has to offer. Being aware or present enhances each and every thing you experience. The power of right NOW is intoxicating and, once you find that moment of space, it feels so pure, like something you have never felt before. It's a little drop of bliss, just like the clarity and vibrancy of a leaf you may have never noticed with those eyes before.

Be aware also of the things you say. Engage your brain before your mouth. Once it's out there, it's too late. When you go to speak, make sure your words are kind, that you speak from your heart's centre, and deliver the words with love. Remember, the energy you put out is what you get back, so be aware; make it good and make it count.

Having an awareness of others around us helps us blend in much better with the many different people we come across during the day. When we become aware of people, we are much more likely to be friendly and say good morning to them. A smile doesn't cost anything and yet it goes such a long way. How many people did you smile at today? Being aware of yourself and how you are feeling will mean that you recognise if you're tense, or stressed or tired. Once you have this awareness, you are more likely to address it rather than ignore how you feel, and less likely to end up snapping at someone because you didn't realise how tired you were, or how hungry you were as you worked through your lunch. When our sugar levels drop, we can become grumpy, irritable or unpleasant to be around, so by being aware of how we are feeling it means we can make the necessary adjustments in order to manage ourselves, by having a drink or some food in this case.

Judgement

Why is it that we judge each other? Why are we so harsh in judging ourselves? Judgement seems such an unkind and unpleasant quality. No one has the right to judge another person. That's where the saying "don't throw stones if you live in a glass house" comes from. It's a good saying to remember and live by. To judge another person is certainly not the way to help you reach your bliss. Instead, pay attention to the words you use when you refer to or talk about others, and also yourself. Celebrate the success of others around you; don't be jealous. Notice the thoughts you think and ensure they are not based on judgement. Instead, be happy for your neighbour's success, new job or new car. Be grateful and celebrate what others have and how well they are doing. Notice and be grateful for your own abundance. Where in your life is there abundance? You may have a wonderful family, a gorgeous home, success in business or fantastic health. When you focus on what you have, you will attract more of the same into your life. When you behave and live from a point of non-judgement, and thankfulness for what you already have, abundance will come into your life in ways you never imagined.

Be sure not to judge other people because, when you judge others, you are actually judging yourself. Every one of us is different; that's what makes life so interesting and people so fascinating. We are all doing the best we can at any given moment with what we know at the time. When you stop judging yourself and other people, you are more able to appreciate the good qualities they have instead. Appreciation is the opposite of judgement, so make sure that you appreciate yourself or someone else every day. Be grateful for what you have, and for the world around you. When you are filled with gratitude, fear disappears. Make your life full of gratitude and appreciation today.

Mindfulness

Inner work is so important and yet here in the western world, many of us have forgotten the importance of integrating mindfulness into our lives. We are not taught the benefits of leading a life of stillness and calm. Yoga, meditation and holistic therapies are around, but not mainstream. Truly connecting with one another is a skill that is not taught in the home, or if it is, it is in the minority of homes. Allowing peace into your life and being in the habit of making the mundane amazing are things we do not practice on the whole. Focusing on the now and being present to this very moment simply doesn't make sense to how we see the world. Instead we rush around at breakneck speed, focusing on the end goal, worrying and stressing that someone else will get there first or that we might fail in some way. We end up missing out on the only true power we have, this very moment. When you put your attention on what you are doing, when you focus on the now, when you decide to enjoy whatever you do, the magic begins to unfold.

You can practice being present in this very moment, and surround yourself with love. Build a deflector shield around you as a protection against hurtful people and unkind words. Remember to let it down with everyone else. Build up your resilience levels so you are ready to face life's challenges head on. By building your resilience levels, you learn to bounce back more quickly when times are hard. At work or home you may encounter people who press your buttons or challenge you in some way, so have a colourful imaginary deflector shield to guard against unkindness. You can visualise it in your favourite colour, or as a bell jar that covers you and protects you from hurtful words.

Over time you will become much more conscious and aware of the damage the ego can cause. The ego is dysfunctional and behaves like a spoilt brat, sabotaging any area of your life and getting attention like an errant child might. Don't let it steal your power and ruin your life. Learn to create flow in your life. Imagine you are the gentle running water trickling down the stream, never stopping, gently caressing the rocks and joining the wider river at its end. Remember how water flows smoothly and slowly. Make sure that you are not rigid like the ice, that's cold, hard and unforgiving. When you behave in a rigid or stubborn way, just like the ice, you too will feel the force as it crashes when hitting a rock and smashes into a thousand pieces. Learn to breathe with an enormous appreciation for the life-giving air that fills your lungs. Breathe slowly in a measured way, from your stomach. Watch it rise and fall with each breath. As you slow down and deepen your breath, relax each part of your body. You can do this on your chair, lying down or even on the train, bus or plane. Never close your eyes whilst driving though. In a very short space of time, you can relax the whole of your body. This is hugely helpful with the crazy lives we all lead. You need only spend 10 minutes in the morning and 10 minutes in the afternoon to stop, sit down, and close your eyes and breathe in and out, slowly, at your own pace. You can breathe in and count if that helps to distract you, or you can take 3 deep breaths and imagine you are on the most beautiful, warm and sandy beach, imagine that the sound of the waves are close by and the wind is gently rustling the leaves on the trees. Imagine you are on your own, with the blue sky up above and the sand below is holding you. You feel safe, and secure. You are at peace and your mind is clear. You feel completely relaxed and blessed. This is your space.

You can try a body scan during your day to check in and see how tense you are. When you take the time to check in, so to speak, you start to notice that you may be more uptight than you thought. Once you recognise this you can begin to relax. This is an easy way of scanning your whole body from your head to your toes. At each part of your body, you notice whether you are feeling a little tense and breathe in and out slowly as you relax that part of your body. This is especially helpful for those of you who work at the computer, where your shoulders and back are more likely to build tension throughout the day.
Mindfulness is extremely effective at managing anxiety and stress. As you all know, stress is everywhere, and can be damaging when left unchecked. By following regular practices

of mindfulness you can overcome anxiety, panic attacks and stress. You could look at it as a tool to help you through the day. Others will also notice how much more relaxed you are when you become regularly mindful. Your energy shifts and changes. You may notice that you start to attract different kinds of people into your life. These people will be attracted to you by your energy. Those with positive energy and calmness will attract similar sorts of people. You may find that your life starts to get a little easier. You might feel lighter, perhaps even younger as you learn to lift the weight of the world off your shoulders.

Mindfulness is starting to be recognised as a helpful tool in schools, hospitals and also in the treatment of patients with psychological problems. It aids with concentration and so helps children to learn, particularly those who naturally become distracted. It calms the mind and so is extremely effective at calming troubled, angry or aggressive children. It's empowering too, because in easy steps children can be taught these techniques. Once they learn ways to become mindful, they can practice at home, or anywhere else. It is a great mechanism to help you cope when you are feeling scared or down.

Meditation

There are many ways to meditate. It's best to choose the one that feels the most comfortable to you. You can use a brief meditation in bed before you get up. You are already relaxed, lying down with your eyes closed, so it's really easy. Take a few deep breaths. You can place your hand on your solar plexus (the stomach area) to focus your mind on the gentle rise and fall of your stomach as you breathe. You can also do a short meditation at bedtime before you sleep. It helps calm the mind and prepare your body for a relaxing and peaceful sleep. After about three deep controlled breaths, imagine that you are in a lush green pasture, the sky is blue and you are under your favourite tree. The sun is warm and the air is still. This is a beautiful mediation for connection with all things. Imagine with each breath that you take, every child, woman and man is breathing in with you. Feel the power of that connection. Feel the clean, fresh air filling your lungs, reaching every cell in your body, feeding your brain. As you breathe out, let go of all of the negative thoughts that may be still in your head. Release any feelings that no longer serve you and relax.

Feel the connection that this powerful meditation brings out of the connection with all of mankind, feel the energy, and feel the strength. Imagine you are breathing with all the animals; you share the same air, they feel your power and you feel theirs. Feel the solidness of mother earth and feel this connection. Let it flow through your whole being. Allow yourself to be in this moment, to feel secure, connected and loved.

There are many meditations for you to find the one that resonates with you. You can meditate anywhere and it's free. You can meditate in a group if you are unsure of what to do. At first it might feel a little strange, especially if you have never meditated before. The important thing is to do a little at a time, each day. Meditation re-energises you, balances you, and is immensely powerful. When you take a few minutes each day to become mindful, do a quick body scan or meditate, you will find your inner strength increase and your health improves.

EFT

This is a technique also known as "tapping" that is quick and easy to teach and very easy to follow yourself. Emotional Freedom Technique is a powerful therapy that works much more quickly than the more traditional therapies. It looks at how the beliefs, habits and prejudices you carry with you from your childhood affect your life as you enter adulthood. The decisions you subconsciously make in childhood are carried through to your life as a grown-up. Some of these thoughts or beliefs no longer serve us and need to be tapped into and let go of. EFT can help with curing addictions and bad habits. Tapping helps to focus you, so public speakers sometimes use it before they go on stage to calm their nerves and keep them on the ball. Many elite athletes use this technique to focus them on their sport, particularly before a race or competition. The beauty of EFT is that, once taught, you can practice it on yourself. It is safe and easy to follow, even for children. Once you learn how to apply this technique, it can be used anywhere and by anyone.

New Daily Rituals

Here is a Body Scan that can help relax you when you are a bit uptight. You can use it in the morning by working from the toes up to the head. This brings the energy up through your body and energises you for the day.

At the end of the day, repeat this exercise except that this time we are taking the energy down and so you start off with the top of the head and work your way down to your feet.

Follow this process a few times. It takes only a couple of minutes.

When you adopt this routine in the morning, as soon as you wake up and before you jump out of bed, it will set you up and ground you for the rest of your day.

Now we will start. Make sure you are lying down for this, or you can sit if you want to give yourself a midday boost.

When you carry out your body scan in a sedentary position, ensure your feet are firmly flat on the floor. This will help to root you.

When you can do this before you get out of bed, you will already have your eyes closed and be relaxed.

Take three deep breaths, to get you ready and relax your whole body.

As you take these deep breaths, completely relax your body as you breathe out. Make sure you are comfortable.

In your mind's eye, visualise your toes, then your feet, the soles of your feet, your arches, the heels of your feet then your ankles, you calves and shins, your knees.

Move onto your thighs, your pelvis and hips, the bottom of your spine.

Scan your fingers, hands wrists and forearms. Focus on your elbows and the tops of your arms.

See your lower back, stomach, upper back and torso.

Then move to your shoulder and neck, relaxing each part of your body as you go.

Relax your jaw, chin, mouth, cheeks, nose, ears, eyes, eye brows and forehead.

Totally relax the back of your head and the top of your head. Repeat this between three and five times.

See how you feel. (If you are seated, make sure you feel supported.) This is a body scan of your whole body, from your toes to your head.

Carry out the exercise in reverse when you want to wind down at the end of the day and start with your head, moving down to your toes.

Imagine you are calming the energy in your body at the end of the day.

This will leave you feeling peaceful and relaxed and help you to sleep more deeply and peacefully.

Chapter 10
Take Full Responsibility For Your Life

The best time to plant a tree was 20 years ago.
The second best time is now.
– Chinese Proverb

Take 100% Responsibility For Everything In Your Life Through Love

Learn to love yourself. Become completely responsible for loving yourself. Surround yourself with a loving environment; bring love into your work and your home. Take a few minutes once a week to spread love into each and every room of your home, and to nurture and love yourself and those you care for. Each morning as you travel to work, bless the road, your car, other people around you, the approach to work, the carpark, the entrance and your office. You can even bless your desk, computer, phone and your colleagues. Because love is a powerful energy, by blessing everything around you, you are raising the vibrations to a positive state that will fill you up. It will also raise the vibration of those around you and fill them up too.

It is not the responsibility of someone else to come along and make you happy. If you think like that, then you will be deeply disappointed and disillusioned. For years, I waited around for my prince charming to show up, and the fact was that every time

I thought I met him and gave him the responsibility to make me happy, he never did. The reason for that was that it wasn't his job to make me happy; it was mine. And for four decades I held this very limiting view. Well I have news for you, for little girls reading nursery rhymes that teach such nonsense this view can be quite damaging. The reason for this is that you are responsible for your own happiness and everything else in your life. Once I discovered that for myself, I felt so much freer, I felt invigorated, that I could chose to make myself happy. Wow! What a discovery.

Winning isn't everything, but wanting to win is.
–Vince Lombardi

It isn't having all the material possessions around you that make you happy either; it is the inner peace of knowing who you are and embracing that, that gives you a really deep sense of happiness and joy. It is being able to share all the good things in your life with other people that brings you happiness.

When we find our Bliss, we become more peaceful and serene. This is mainly because we have learned to not worry, as it's such a waste of our energy, and we have come to trust that the universe is here to hold us all and that life is a series of lessons to help us learn and grow. And best of all, life is an adventure and, just like at a fairground, we can choose which rides we want to go on. Try them all if you like.

To be loving, kind and compassionate is to treat others as an equal to ourself. We need to accept that, in order for us to grow, we need one another to stretch and at times challenge us along the way. When we truly care for ourselves, we find it much easier to care for each other.

When you gain an understanding that all beings depend on one another and that we are all connected to nature, mother earth and all things, the need to behave in a self-centred way disappears. For we realise that we are no longer separate from each other but connected, and that is our strength. Remember that we rely on the plants to feed us and give us medicines to cure us. The animals feed us and give us milk, cheese, eggs, meat; and fur and leather to cloth us. The trees emit oxygen which maintains our very existence, and they need carbon dioxide to survive, which is what we discard when we breathe out what we no longer need. We completely rely on wood and coal to burn in order for us to stay warm during the colder months, we use wood from the trees to build our homes and create beautiful furniture and toys for our children. We don't need to look far to realise that we are in fact co-dependent on each other and on nature. From time to time it helps to be reminded of everything that we sometimes forget to be grateful for.

Once our emotional state becomes more stable, our ego will begin to fade away. Our ability to show compassion to others will increase and we will feel more peace and harmony in our life. When we feel peaceful, everyone else around us will pick up on this and feel calm in our company.

Practice patience and understanding every day. At first this will test even the most tolerant of you, but in time you will see that when you are patient, you become non-judgemental and the world opens up to you. When you show understanding towards other people, they will open up too, and you will have better relationships in your life.

By adopting a more humble stance in the world, we stand strong and know who we are. We no longer need to have the validation of others in order for us to feel we are someone. We can be open and gentle, and always chose kindness over the need to be right. Embrace the fact that, now that you are realising your Bliss, you are becoming more insightful and open-minded. When we develop an open mind, the world around us has more clarity. We become more accepting and don't jump to conclusions until all is revealed to us. We can develop having a mind that is open to everything and yet at the same time attached to nothing in the material world. It is through attachment that we create insecurities with things and people that we can't take with us. So by learning to let go and de-clutter our homes, garages and offices on a regular basis, we keep our mind de-cluttered too.

Realise your inner strength that is maintained by connecting to nature and all things. The strength that is found through practicing mindfulness and giving yourself space to just be every day, is one way to relieve the tension that builds up in our bodies each day.

Part of taking responsibility for yourself is to lead by example, and to help other people free themselves from the suffering in the world, so that they may benefit from your wisdom and experience. Their suffering might be some small thing like crossing the road at night or asking if they can take a turn at going on their lunch break first. Not everyone is strong, and some people need a little more encouragement than others. By leading the way, others will follow when you set good examples and spread kindness along the way. Why not take in some homemade cakes to work and share them? Or you could offer to buy someone a coffee whom you've never spoken with before.

Ananda – Bliss

Once you have started to do your inner work, you will begin to truly find your Bliss. By taking full and total responsibility for all areas of your life, you will start to see that you have far more control over the direction your life is heading in. This feeling of empowering yourself is very encouraging.

> *Life isn't about getting and having, it's about giving and being.*
> –Kevin Kruse

Take 100% Responsibility For Everything In Your Life Through Acceptance

When we really and truly learn to accept ourselves and others, we take responsibility for who we are. We take the pressure off ourselves to be what we are not. When we end the conflict of trying to be what someone else expects of us, life just starts to feel a little easier. Acceptance creates in us emotional ease and wellbeing.

When you are unable to accept the unknown or uncertainty, you become filled with fear. However, the unknown or uncertainty becomes an adventure when you do accept it. In essence, the outcome of the situation depends entirely on your perception of it.

When you don't accept a situation, you may be filled with fear. However, when you do accept a situation, you become tolerant of it.

When another person hurts you and you are unable to accept this, you are filled with anger and hatred towards that person. However, the minute you can bring yourself to accept this, you become a forgiving person. You also become someone who doesn't carry resentment and therefore lives a lighter life. Your burdens become less when you can accept the hurt others cause you, without feeling waves of hatred towards them. This is called forgiveness and it will set you free.

Have you ever found yourself feeling jealous of someone else, about either who they are or what they have or what they have achieved? When we are jealous of someone else, it means that we have not accepted something as being fair or just in our minds. On the flip side, when we accept and delight in other people's achievements, they become beacons for us. They inspire us to want to pick up the mantle and we can aim to also strive to achieve what our heart desires in our own lives. So once again, when we are in a state of acceptance, we are much more able to achieve what we want in our lives than if we don't accept. This level of acceptance is what's known as emotional maturity. It is the ability to rise above the pettiness that often rules us and holds us back.

I've learned that people will forget what you said, people will forget what you did, but people will never forget how you made them feel.
–Maya Angelou

Take 100% Responsibility For Everything In Your Life Through Forgiveness

Forgiveness, as we have already recognised, is really hard to do. However, it is imperative to forgive others around us who have wronged us, as well as to forgive ourselves, for the wrongs we have caused. In order to take full and complete responsibility for our lives we must forgive. To forgive someone else to the point that we believe the wrong never occurred is the deepest and truest form of forgiveness. Unless we can learn to forgive, we will always become trapped in a world that feels unjust. When we don't forgive, we carry that burden through our life and it becomes a dis-ease in our mind and our body.

When you hold onto resentment, your body tightens up each time you revisit the experience and, unless you can release it, your body will hold onto this forever. You can try this at any time to see how it works. The next time you think of an uncomfortable situation, or a time when someone said something really hurtful towards you, notice how your body feels. Your shoulders may become tense, you may clench your jaw, or you might tighten your fists. You may even stop breathing for a moment, or adopt very shallow breaths. These are all signs of your body carrying the tension from those experiences. Now that you recognise how that feels for you, you can decide what to do about it. Take responsibility for yourself and let these negative feelings go. You can let go of tension by breathing in deeply from the stomach and then as you breathe out, imagine you are releasing all the negative feelings and tension in your whole body. If it helps you focus, place your hand gently on your stomach and feel it expand and contract with your every breath.

Life shrinks or expands in proportion to one's courage.
–Anais Nin

For more tips and easy techniques to help you manage tension and stress visit www.getblissed.com

Take 100% Responsibility For Everything In Your Life By Not Worrying Or Criticising Any More. Ditch The Excuses

We now know that worrying is a completely pointless manmade emotion or feeling. When you worry about something or someone, it puts you in a position of helplessness. You cannot achieve anything through worrying; it's such a total waste of time and energy. If you thought that you only had a certain amount of energy each day, each week or even in your life time, wouldn't you be more careful of how you used it? Of course you would. So let's assume that your energy is limited. This being so, what would you remove from your life? You would probably decide to never worry ever again, because you cannot achieve anything through worrying; it only wastes your energy and puts you in an unhelpful and vulnerable state, a state of helplessness.

You miss 100% of the shots you don't take.
–Wayne Gretzky

When you worry about something that's already happened, there is nothing in the world you can do about it, except accept it and move on. Learn from your mistakes if that's what's bothering you. There are not really any mistakes, just lessons to learn. Why would you want to worry about something in the future? How can you possibly affect something that hasn't happened or that you are fearful of that may or may not happen? Why bother tarnishing this present moment by a situation that may never occur? If you are concerned, then you have two choices, accept what is going to pass, or take action to change it. It really is as simple as that. And yet we continue to make our lives so complicated when they really don't need to be.

Twenty years from now you will be more disappointed by the things that you didn't do than by the ones you did do, so throw off the bowlines, sail away from safe harbor, catch the trade winds in your sails. Explore, Dream, Discover.
–Mark Twain

As we are all connected, when you criticise another person, you are hurting them and yourself. You are also not accepting who they are. As we are all different, what gives any of us the right to criticise another person? This is why criticism is pointless, and yet we all do it. But why? It is because we think we are better or that we know more than the other person, and we act as though we are God. It would be good to remember not to throw stones when we all live in glass houses. When you learn to ignore the ego in your head that says unkind things and criticises, you will feel much better. Remember that together we achieve more than if we act alone.

The most common way people give up their power is by thinking they don't have any.
—Alice Walker

You will meet the "Excuse" people from time to time. These are the people that will do this when they get time, or do that when they get a day off. In fact if you watch them closely, they don't ever get around to doing anything that they said they will. That's fine for them, if they are happy plodding along, except that when they get to the end of their lives, it won't be the things they did that they will regret doing, but the things they didn't.

The two most important days in your life are the day you are born and the day you find out why.
—Mark Twain

Ultimately, it's up to you what your life looks like; it is, after all, YOUR life. Whatever you want your life to look like, whatever you can dream up, whatever you can conceive, when you attach a strong consistent positive emotion to that thought and think it with all your might and each day take a small step towards that goal, eventually you will reach it. You really cannot fail. I'll prove it. If you are over there and you want to come over here, all you have to do is start to take small steps towards me over here. Then in a very short space of time, you will arrive from over there to over here, next to me, see? There you go; you did it. Simple, well done.

I attribute my success to this: I never gave or took any excuse.
 −Florence Nightingale

Take 100% Responsibility For Everything In Your Life Through Affirmations and Thoughts To Support and Maintain You

The mind is everything. What you think you become.
−Buddha

To stop the chatter in your head, or the monkey mind as Buddhists call it, you can focus fully on the present moment. Pay attention to what you are doing right now. You can take a metaphorical step back and simply observe the thoughts in your head without engaging with them, or you can say affirmations to support a positive state of mind for yourself. When we use affirmations to improve our thoughts, quiet our mind or to keep us focused, for each one of us, the affirmations will be different. You can say anything that you like that positively reinforces the direction you wish to go in. Whether you want to buy your first home, look for a new job, have your health back, come first in a race, or receive the biggest bonus in your company, once you believe you can and imagine that you will, you can use affirmations to support whatever is important for you. For example you could say "Thank you for this amazing day I am having" or if you are in a difficult situation at work you might repeat in your head "I am patient and resilient" or "I only speak words of love." These are just a couple of examples to show you that, whatever you say, it needs to be positive, in the present and relevant to you at this very moment.

Strive not to be a success, but rather to be of value.
−Albert Einstein

When you are present, and in this moment, you notice everything around you in much more detail. So for example, whilst I am typing, I notice the sound of my fingers clicking on the keys, I notice the dull hum of the traffic in the background as it drives by outside, the noisy zoom of the moped that just sped by, the quiet, regular rumble of the fridge and the dripping of the water through the fish tank. If I pay even more attention, I become aware of my breathing. Once I bring my attention to my breathing, I actually consciously maintain a deep and regular in and out of my breath. I noticed that the breath was more shallow when I first brought my attention to it than I would prefer, so I regulate it accordingly. Now I mindfully breathe fully into my stomach, then fill up my lungs, before releasing the air again, along with the tension that's built up in my shoulders as I type.

We become what we think about.
–Earl Nightingale

Our thoughts are powerful; they create the future for us. Be sure to keep your thoughts positive. In order to take full responsibility for everything in your life you will need to make sure that everything you read, think and say supports the direction you want to go. So, on a daily basis, it does mean being mindful and aware of what you think and say. It is easier to keep under control what you read, as there are many books to help with this. Also, when you do read you become engrossed with your book, giving it your full attention. Whether you choose self-help books or books to educate yourself, there is information everywhere, in the library, on the book shelf, information on your computer, your laptop or even your phone. In fact, in today's society with information at our very finger tips 24/7, it's the easiest time to educate ourselves.

Whatever the mind of man can conceive and believe, it can achieve.
–Napoleon Hill

Take 100% Responsibility For Everything In Your Life Through Taking Care Of Your Body, Mind and Soul

You attract everything that happens to your body. Take the time to relax at least twice a day, to unwind and release the tension that has built up over the course of your day.

Eighty percent of success is showing up.
–Woody Allen

You need to be mindful of your physical, emotional and mental health, and keep it in harmony. Have fun eating and drinking only healthy foods and drinks. Learn how to blend yourself a delicious smoothie with fresh or frozen fruits and natural yoghurt and local, runny honey. Why not juice some greens, celery, apples and fresh mint along with plenty of clean water? Then see how great your body feels with all that goodness inside of you. Once you start to honour yourself and really take care of your body, wanting to keep fit and exercise will feel natural to you and become second nature. Make sure that you do what makes you feel good; it shouldn't be an effort. Each morning when you awaken, take a moment to be truly grateful for the brand new day that lies ahead of you. Each and every day is a new opportunity to start over. Start your day with just ten minutes of a simple breathing mindful exercise or a meditation. Do your affirmations throughout the day to quiet the chatter in your mind. Say helpful affirmations in your head throughout the day like "I love and approve of myself" or "I am valued by my colleagues" or "My boss notices how hard I'm working and rewards me."

Every strike brings me closer to the next home run.
—Babe Ruth

Be kind to yourself. Realise and acknowledge that we are all doing the best we can with what we know at this exact moment in time. When you feel as though you haven't achieved as much as you would have liked to, congratulate yourself for getting this far and achieving all the things you have. It is when we look back rather than forward that we can see where we have come so far. Then we can be grateful for all our accomplishments.

You can never cross the ocean until you have the courage to lose sight of the shore.
—Christopher Columbus

Remember to honour your spiritual practice daily to maintain your balance. As in all things, maintenance is crucial to keep a healthy spiritual state. And so to meditate and carry out mindfulness practices, do yoga or the equivalent is essential for a healthy mind. It is so easy to neglect ourselves with the hustle and bustle of our demanding daily lives.

Whether you think you can or you think you can't, you're right.
—Henry Ford

Take 100% Responsibility For Everything In Your Life Through Educating Yourself

We all go to school to receive an education; it's what we have to do. It's the bare minimum and we think that's all the education we will need. Then some of us go on to college or university. Once we leave the education system and find a job for ourselves, we often forget that the education continues only if we want it to. I remember leaving school and then leaving college and thinking to myself, wow, thank goodness for that, no more learning for me. I can get on with my life. Little did I know how naive that statement would turn out to be for me.

> *Your time is limited, so don't waste it living someone else's life.*
> –Steve Jobs

Now that I am older and hopefully a little wiser, I see the world very differently. The more I learn, the more I realise I don't know. Nowadays, I absolutely love learning new things. I feel like a sponge and want to learn something new every day. In fact I did go back to take my degree 11 years after leaving college for the second time. It was really tough for me and I was the oldest student in my class, but I was ready for a new challenge and thoroughly enjoyed student life in my late twenties. Several years ago I took a marketing course, which was most informative and now I am ready for another new challenge. So in my experience, the learning has been ongoing. For those who leave school and never go back, life is your education, and Lord Sugar has proved that when you are hard-working and have the focus and dedication to succeed, you can achieve anything you want. All you need is to believe in yourself.

> *Whatever you can do, or dream you can, begin it.*
> *Boldness has genius, power and magic in it.*
> –Johann Wolfgang von Goethe

My children have been my most surprising teachers, but teachers they are, nevertheless. There is an old proverb that says, when you're ready to learn, your teacher will appear. I believe that to be true and from my perspective feel blessed to have had so many teachers sign-posting me along the way. Courses, people and books have shown up in my life at just the right time and in the most bizarre ways. One book has led to me meeting someone and then someone recommended a book, and then a course presented itself to me and before I knew it, all the dots started to join up. The crazy thing is that it's only as I look back that I can see where all the dots were heading. When I was looking ahead, the path wasn't clear further than a couple of steps ahead of me. These days I have learned to trust that's what life looks like, when you believe and trust.

People often say that motivation doesn't last. Well, neither does bathing. That's why we recommend it daily.
–Zig Ziglar

Take 100% Responsibility For Everything In Your Life Through Only Watching and Reading Positive Things

The mind is a powerful entity. It sits outside of our physical being and keeps records of everything. Based on our perspective on life, we readily recall what resonates with us. The mind cannot distinguish between a dream and a memory. The mind processes dreams in the same way as it does real and actual experiences. By the same token, the films we watch at the movies and on the television have an effect on us too. For me, if I watch a thriller, I will physically start to shake at the scary parts. My body is reacting as though I was right there in the movie. So, if like me, you react like this, be careful what you watch. Now that I am aware of this and recognise that I am sensitive in this way, I choose not to watch thrillers. Instead I love nature programmes or documentaries or well-written comedies, or sometimes period dramas. Also I never watch soap operas, as I find they bring my mood down.

Life is 10% what happens to me and 90% of how I react to it.
–Charles Swindoll

Of course, each one of us is different and as long as you can watch something without being affected in a similar way to me, by all means go ahead. The thing is though, that when we watch the news with all its doom and gloom and violence, even though we may think it has no effect on us, the mind still processes this information. When we watch anything of a violent nature, the more anger, frustration, irritation and other such senses are aroused in us. When we are continuously exposed to such things, our memory lessens, our immune system depletes and our heart contracts. At the same time, when we watch funny programmes, stand-up comedy or films about the world and nature, painted in the positive, our hearts open, our minds expand and our wellbeing improves. Even our memories sharpen when we smile and laugh, and so does our immune system.

Either you run the day, or the day runs you.
–Jim Rohn

When you wake up in the morning and when you go to sleep at night, you want to be able to set the scene for the next 8-10 hours. So it makes sense in the morning when you wake up, to be grateful for the new day ahead. Decide to be happy at the fact that you are alive. You can look forward to your day and the opportunity to learn new things, or whatever it is that feels good for you. It may be looking forward to a meal out with friends at the end of the day that makes you smile; it could be a trip to the gym after work, a lunchtime date with an old friend, or an interview for a brand new job. Whatever it is, when it's in the positive (feelings of love, joy, peace, abundance, happiness, passion, light), it sets you up for the day. If you get out of bed and stub your toe, then swear at the rain outside, this is how you will set yourself up for the day. So the choice is yours. Make the start of your day count. It's your life.

Get Blissed

> *I am not a product of my circumstances.*
> *I am a product of my decisions.*
> –Stephen Covey

At the end of the day, your brain is going to get between 6-8 hours of sleep to work its magic on you, so go to bed feeling great about what you have achieved that day. You may like to do some exercise in the evening or go for a walk to tire your body out, and get ready for sleep. You may prefer to meditate to calm your mind down. It is preferable not to watch the television or have any screen time just before you go to bed as your brain waves won't be ready to sleep if you do.

What do you like to read? Do you enjoy fiction, non-fiction, poetry, history, biographies, newspapers or something else? What we read defines us. The books we read influence how we see the world; they expand our view or contract it, depending on the subject matter. Do you like to learn new things? Are you fixated by the same author? Are you fascinated by machinery, space, engineering?

> *The most difficult thing is the decision to act,*
> *the rest is merely tenacity.*
> –Amelia Earhart

Take 100% Responsibility For Everything In Your Life Through Awareness Of Everything and Everyone Around You

> *An unexamined life is not worth living.*
> –Socrates

Conclusion

It's Up To You

Once you fully embrace who you are, you might feel that you don't want to be part of the herd any more. You might find that being like marmite suits you; some love you, whilst others just don't seem to get you. That's fine! You can't please everyone, so why use up your energy trying? Once you have broken through the chaos in your life and in your head, you start to expand and become the magnificent being you were always meant to be. Your inner beauty will begin to shine through as you unfold into a bright light, that gets reflected in every area of your life. As a by-product of this transformation, you will find that, in order for you to be so right for some people, you inadvertently become so wrong for others.

Definiteness of purpose is the starting point of all achievement.
–W. Clement Stone

Never be afraid to indulge in what makes your heart sing, what helps your creativity to grow and flow. Be prepared to regularly push the boundaries and step outside of your comfort zone. Feel how alive running in a hail storm makes you; the adrenalin and rush of air passing over your whole body when you sky dive; the nerves you experience when you sing for the first time at a karaoke just because it's what you feel like doing inside. Never allow the judgement of others to hold you back.

Life is about making an impact, not making an income.
—Kevin Kruse

When you need to get back your power, to get clarity and take charge of a situation, go for a walk; it's really effective. Treat yourself to a walk in the morning, at lunchtime, or in the middle of the night; it's exhilarating. Ironically sitting at your desk won't help the creative juices flow and so getting out and having a change of scenery is much better. If this really isn't possible, use a white board to scribble down what's in your head. If you can find a colleague whose skills complement yours, then even better. Ask for their help. You are taking responsibility for the direction of your creativity and make your working life a liberating experience.

Every child is an artist. The problem is how to remain an artist once he grows up.
—Pablo Picasso

Taking responsibility for yourself means trying, falling over and picking yourself back up again time and time again. It is turning up and never giving up that makes us into winners.

*I've missed more than 9000 shots in my career. I've lost almost 300 games. 26 times I've been trusted to take the game winning shot and missed. I've failed over and over and over again in my life.
And that is why I succeed.*
—Michael Jordan

About the author

Natasha Aylott developed her own unique approach to life that will help you. She has adapted this for mentoring, coaching and workshops. In addition, Natasha is available for motivational sessions and keynote speeches talking about her passion, returning to health and happiness from the inside out.

After nearly a decade of extensive research in the field of spirituality, Natasha has learned, practiced and adopted amazing and easy ways to change your life through changing your thoughts and building love into each and every area of her life. Areas including home life, work life and relationships. Discovering and embracing that life loves you.

Studying psychology, EFT, NLP, CBT alongside spirituality has given Natasha a fantastic insight into finding your Bliss and de-stressing your life. Now well-versed in these areas, Natasha's wish is to share the experience and knowledge she has gained to help others around the globe to step into their own power, take ownership for their lives and live their Bliss.

Natasha's work includes a close affiliation with the charity Mentorlink and Safeline, where she continues to mentor in schools. This approach has been carried over into the workplace and is available in bite-size pieces to blow away the negativity from the playground to the boardroom, within the world of commerce and industry. Natasha happily invites you to share your moments on her Facebook page www.facebook.com/natashaaylott. If you would like to hire her for keynote speeches or workshops or seminars, and for more information, visit www.getblissed.co.uk

Printed in Great Britain
by Amazon.co.uk, Ltd.,
Marston Gate.